Prescription Pot

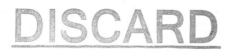

Prescription Pot

*A Leading Advocate's Heroic Battle
to Legalize Medical Marijuana*

By
George McMahon
and Christopher Largen

New Horizon Press
Far Hills, New Jersey

New Horizon Press
P.O. Box 669
Far Hills, NJ 07931

George McMahon and Christopher Largen
    Prescription Pot: A Leading Advocate's Heroic Battle to Legalize Medical
    Marijuana

Cover Design: Mike Stromberg, The Great American Art Company
Interior Design: Susan M. Sanderson

Library of Congress Control Number: 2003105912

ISBN: 0-88282-240-3
New Horizon Press

Manufactured in the U.S.A.

2007   2006   2005   2004   2003   /   5   4   3   2   1

A journey is a person in itself; no two are alike...We find after years of struggle that we do not take a trip; a trip takes us.

– John Steinbeck, *Travels with Charley*

History indicates the most trivial of facts can implode the most powerful dogma.

– Robert Randall, *Marijuana Rx*

health (helth) n. Broadly, any state of optimal functioning, well-being, or progress.

– The American Heritage Dictionary of the English Language

Dedication

I wish to thank my wife Margaret, my mother June, my children Linda, Sean, and Jennifer, my grandkids, all the wonderful people I've met along the green path, Burt, Jeanie, Jody, and finally my little dog Barbie and her pup Tuffy. And thanks to Christopher, the first classic iconoclast I ever met.

  - George McMahon

I extend deep gratitude to my wife Gynni–for her faith, hope, patience, and charity. We laugh through tears; you keep me hanging on.

To mom and dad–for always being there.

To my children Caleb and Liberty–for bringing more joy into my life than I ever deserved. May you grow strong and healthy.

To Nathan–for the crash pad and the munchies

To Elvis–for being my muse

To all patients–for inspiration

To George–for showing me the path

  - Christopher Largen

Table of Contents

Author's Note

This book is based on George McMahon's actual experiences and reflects his perception of the past, present and future. The personalities, events, actions and conversations portrayed within the story have been reconstructed from his memory and the memories of participants. In an effort to safeguard individual privacy, the names of certain people have been changed and, in some cases, otherwise identifying characteristics have been altered. Events involving the characters happened as described; only minor details have been changed.

Foreword

By
Mary Lynn Mathre

Mary Lynn Mathre has worked as a registered nurse in acute care facilities for more than twenty-seven years. From 1987 through 2002 she specialized in addictions nursing at the University of Virginia. She is the editor of Cannabis in Medical Practice: A Legal, Historical and Pharmacological Overview of the Therapeutic Use of Marijuana, *published in 1997 by McFarland & Company. She also serves on the editorial board of the* Journal of Cannabis Therapeutics *published by Haworth Press. Mary Lynn is the president and one of the co-founders of Patients Out of Time.*

I first met George McMahon in 1990, at NORML's (National Organization for the Reform of Marijuana Laws) annual conference in Washington, D.C. George was participating on a panel featuring the first five legal medical marijuana patients in the United States. At the time, I was the Director of NORML's Council on Marijuana and Health and I was also a member of the Board of Directors. My husband, Al Byrne, was also a member of the NORML Board, as well as an officer of the organization. The two of us were responsible for the conference program that year. While we believed that prohibiting the use of marijuana by adults and punishing those who choose to use it is unjust and un-American, we were appalled by the fact that the United States government was actually targeting and arresting patients as criminals. We believed this problem needed more attention, so we established the issue of therapeutic cannabis as a top priority for NORML.

As a registered nurse for twenty-seven years, I felt it was important for the public to hear from patients about the advantages of marijuana usage in certain medical circumstances. Years earlier I had met Robert Randall, the first patient to receive medical marijuana from the United States government. Together with his partner, Alice O'Leary, they founded the Alliance of Cannabis Therapeutics (ACT), the first non-profit organization advocating for patient access to cannabis. With help from Robert and Alice, Al and I contacted the other four patients who legally received medical marijuana and invited them to come to the conference and participate in a panel discussion about their medical use of cannabis. To our delight, they all agreed. Robert Randall came from his home in the capital, Elvy Mussika and Irv Rosenfeld flew in from Florida, Corrine Millet from Nebraska and George McMahon from Iowa. This was the first time these five individuals were all together.

The presentation was powerful. The five men and women spoke the simple truth and their words elicited tears and laughter from the audience. The panelists were authentic and it was clear their suffering was real as they explained how cannabis improved the quality of their lives when conventional medical treatments had failed. Their presentation was taped by C-SPAN and for the next month it was repeatedly aired on national television, allowing this important issue to reach a larger and larger audience. Public awareness of the therapeutic use of cannabis and the legal access to federal marijuana supplies spread throughout the nation. This event precipitated an avalanche of patient applications for medical cannabis through the FDA's Compassionate IND (Investigational New Drug) program.

While staying at the hotel where the conference was held, George and the other patients agreed to be interviewed for the purpose of creating an educational video about therapeutic cannabis. The video would feature the only patients in the United States who openly can talk about their use of medical cannabis without fear of arrest. Videographer, Roger Grant, graciously agreed to film the interviews pro bono and he served as the film's editor to help us teach the public about cannabis through the voices of the government program's participating patients. Other individuals and companies anonymously donated their expertise and technology to the project. *Marijuana as Medicine*, an eighteen-minute video, was completed and released in 1992, and is still used as a teaching aid that often brings viewers to tears.

That same year, the government blocked access to the federal marijuana program for all new and pending patients. By 1992, there were fifteen patients receiving marijuana from the government. More than thirty-two additional patient applications were approved, and about 2000 applications were waiting for review. The federal government feared the Compassionate IND program for medical marijuana was gaining too much attention. How could the government continue an anti-drug campaign about the dangers of marijuana while, at the same time, supply cannabis as medicine for sick people? The federal government coldly informed those patients whose applications for medical marijuana had been approved that they would, in fact, never receive their medicine. Those applications still waiting for review would go unanswered as the federal officials slammed the door shut to the only legal access to cannabis in the United States. George and the other fourteen patients who had been receiving their marijuana before the closure of this program would be the only American citizens allowed to use marijuana legally in the future. George learned with sadness that Ladd Huffman, a fellow Iowa patient who suffers from multiple sclerosis was among the thirty-plus approved patients who would not get the medicine they were promised.

When I first met George, he had only recently been accepted into the IND program and was in a wheelchair much of the time. He could walk short distances only with the help of a wooden cane. His body was beginning to adjust to going without the numerous prescription medications he had been taking before he found medical cannabis. I've been in close contact with him since that first meeting and have watched his health continue to improve. When I drove out to Iowa for a visit with George and his wife, Margaret, in July 2000, he used no wheelchair or cane. He met me at the end of his drive-way on a bicycle and then, riding his bike, he escorted me up the gravel road several hundred yards to his home.

From the first time I met him, George was ready, willing and eager to do his part to help other patients get access to cannabis. Before he owned a computer, George would get on-line at his local library, answering questions from patients and concerned citizens. He would talk to anyone willing to listen and learn about how cannabis helped him. As you will read in this book, he and Margaret traveled thousands of miles across the country on a shoestring budget to speak with citizens and legislators. He made these long trips in the hope that he might make a difference, especially for those denied medical marijuana. Although his wife is camera-shy and quiet, she traveled with him and supported his efforts.

George was with us from the start in 1994 when we developed the concept for our non-profit organization, Patients Out of Time. Years earlier, we had met a sweet young couple from Florida who were outspoken in their advocacy for medical marijuana. Kenny Jenks was a hemophiliac and required periodic transfusions of blood-clotting factors. Unfortunately, one of his transfusions was contaminated with HIV and he became infected. He unknowingly infected his wife Barbara, and the two of them subsequently developed AIDS. The couple was wasting away from the disease when they learned from fellow patients in their AIDS support group that marijuana might stop their violent retching and stimulate their appetites. They gained legal access to medical marijuana before the IND program closed and, despite their poor health, they worked with the Alliance for Cannabis Therapeutics to help other AIDS patients submit IND applications for this medicine. These two compassionate individuals died shortly thereafter from AIDS, and as George and I mourned their deaths, we realized that there would be fewer and fewer Americans left alive who could speak openly about their use of ther-apeutic cannabis without being subject to arrest.

We chose the name, Patients Out of Time, to symbolize the urgent need for change. For countless patients, cannabis is the only medicine that eases their suffering and many have no choice but to break the law in order to gain relief. The cruelty of this prohibition is unforgivable. Patients Out of Time is dedicated to educating public citizens and health care professionals about the therapeutic use of cannabis, with the ultimate goal of placing it back into the pharmacopoeia.

George is one of the co-founders of Patients Out of Time and serves on our Board of Directors. By having George and other patients actively involved, we all stay focused on the urgency of our fight. Cannabis does have therapeutic value, and for some patients it is the only remedy for their suffering. Decreased pain and spasticity, increased appetite, reduced nausea and vomiting, improved mood and stable eyesight are all typical results associated with the use of this medicine. Cannabis undoubtedly helps with a wide variety of symptoms for patients with different diseases or conditions.

In May 2001, my husband Al and I traveled from Virginia to Missoula, Montana to meet with three of the legal medical patients. Our purpose was to conduct an intensive study of the chronic effects of cannabis on these government supplied marijuana patients. George and Margaret drove up from Texas while the other two patients flew in from out-of-state to be a part of the Missoula Chronic Use Study. A fourth patient who was unable to travel the distance, participated in the study by having the same tests done locally. The study was designed and led by Ethan Russo, M.D., a Missoula-based neurologist they trusted and respected.

For the next three days, these patients consented to various exams and tests. The hospital staff was empathetic and the patients' testing schedules allowed for necessary rest periods and medication breaks. All went smoothly until it was time for George to allow a technician to draw his blood. Years ago, George had decided he would not have any more blood taken from him. He had experienced far too many needles throughout his life and he finally called it quits. It was his decision and none of us felt we had any right to pressure him. Relieved that he could have his way on this issue,

George considered the fact that there would be some missing information in the final results. Before it was too late, he changed his mind and allowed the blood work. His commitment to the study was more important to him than his personal qualms.

These patients had been using a known dosage of quality-controlled cannabis on a daily basis for eleven to twenty-seven years, certainly long enough to demonstrate any possible adverse effects. The study team thought a thorough examination of the chronic effects of marijuana would be of immense value. We wondered why the government continued to report negative long-term effects of marijuana, yet never conducted such a study on the patients whose medicine they were supplying.

George is someone who understands what it means to live with pain and suffering. He knows how cruel and unfair it is that he gets his medicine from the federal government, yet countless other patients (including his own children), have no legal access. George is one of my heroes. He chooses to speak out against the unjust prohibition of medical marijuana, even at the risk of having the government take his medicine away from him. He willingly allowed highly personal medical information to be released to the public through the Missoula Chronic Use study. Although we tried to report the findings in a manner that would protect his privacy, it is apparent that patient B is George—the patient with the rare genetic disorder called Nail-Patella syndrome.

In 1999, per the request of the Director of the Office of National Drug Control Policy (ONDCP), the Institute of Medicine (IOM) completed an eighteen-month study to evaluate the science behind the therapeutic use of cannabis. Published as *Marijuana and Medicine: Assessing the Science Base* (National Academy Press, 1999), the study concluded that marijuana does have therapeutic value, but government officials engaged in a "war on drugs" have ignored or denied the study's conclusions and recommendations. Since then, the governments of several European countries, Canada and other nations have recognized the therapeutic value of cannabis and further clinical trials are supporting its efficacy. Not only have United States federal officials ignored the IOM study, but they have also displayed a bias of ethnocentricity by totally ignoring the combined science of the world regarding therapeutic cannabis.

Our federal government remains firmly committed to prohibition and recently the Drug Enforcement Agency (DEA) has focused much of its resources on targeting medical marijuana patients and those who grow marijuana for patients. Politicians and DEA officials continue promoting the absurd notion that those who support legalization of medical marijuana—"legalizers"—are simply using patients to get legal access to marijuana. They charge that legalizers are playing a "cruel hoax" on patients by falsely claiming that marijuana is medicine.

I served four years of active duty as an officer in the United States Navy Nurse Corps and my husband is a twenty-year veteran U.S. Naval officer who has served in combat. We understand the rules of war and we know the federal government has waged a war on drugs (drug users). However, the ill treatment of the wounded (patients) is the worst demonstration of mendacity and barbarism in warfare. The official policy of the United States government vilifies the wounded. The government accuses patients of using their suffering as a means to ensure that strangers in their midsts can "get high."

Like them, even George McMahon was once mistaken about the therapeutic value of cannabis. Before using therapeutic cannabis, his life consisted of multiple hospitalizations, thousands of doses of prescription medicines with intense, debilitating side effects, being bedridden for long periods and requiring the use of a wheelchair, a cane and various body splints. Since smoking cannabis on a regular basis, he hasn't been hospitalized, he is off all other medications, he drives around the country, he is able to walk with just a cane and often has a smile on his face. He still suffers from awful symptoms and he does not have much endurance, but with cannabis he has a **better life**! The cruel hoax is that the federal government does not care about other suffering patients who could experience similar benefits if allowed to participate in the IND program.

As a registered nurse, I've cared for countless patients with debilitating or life-threatening illnesses. I've learned that all medications come with risks and even the most "highly recommended" medications may cause adverse reactions, including death. I've learned that in order to give the best care to my patients, I need to listen to them. I need to observe their responses to various treatments and medications. George's experience with therapeutic cannabis is clearly an example of good medicine: highly beneficial with minimal risks. This is the goal for all health care professionals—to provide treatments that will improve a patient's condition without adding unwanted side effects or adverse consequences.

Therapeutic cannabis has improved the quality of life for George as well as the six other surviving legal patients. That's right, only seven of the fifteen federally supplied medical marijuana patients are still alive today. Of them, only four dare to speak openly about its benefits. On behalf of Patients Out of Time, I hope that the green path will soon be open to the innumerable individuals who are currently patients running out of time.

Introduction

In 1990, the year George McMahon first received marijuana from the federal government's Compassionate Investigational New Drug (IND) program, I had no idea that I would become personally involved in the issue of medical cannabis. In fact, it was an issue I knew little about. Living in Ft. Worth, Texas, like many young adults of limited means, I was sweating my way through college, banging my aching head against a monolithic and seemingly insurmountable ivory tower.

I lived frugally, making a conscious effort to cultivate a lifestyle of material austerity. My mind was full, if not my stomach. When my pantry was depleted I would dine cerebrally, devouring the works of Fyodor Dostoyevski, Franz Kafka, William Shakespeare and Stephen King. I switched to a vegetarian diet, clipped coupons and read by candlelight. Anything to make ends meet. Still, someone had to bring home the tofu.

I finally took a job as a personal care attendant for Roy, a quadriplegic Vietnam veteran who had been shot in the back. For more than a year I worked closely with him, seven days a week, morning and night. I helped him bathe and dress, I changed his bedpans and I listened to his sorrows, trying my best to empathize with a terrible situation I could only begin to understand.

1

In time, I became keenly aware of how many precious gifts I had taken for granted in my life. It wasn't that I felt some misplaced sense of guilt about the fact that Roy was paralyzed from his chest down, but I did regret that I had not previously appreciated the simple functionality of my own body. After all, I could still feel the green grass between my toes, ride a bicycle and jump in the ocean on a starry night.

The essential process of self-discovery and rehabilitative transition following a spinal-cord injury is inevitably challenging, but for Roy the basic struggle of daily life was excruciating. His positive self-esteem was dependent upon his independence, yet he required assistance in virtually every aspect of his life.

He suffered from intense depression, haunted by the notion that the person he once was no longer existed. He was once a soldier, but now he was unable to control his own bowels. His desperate situation was compounded by vicious spasms that began in his atrophied legs, crept up his back and seized his entire body in a violent paroxysm of agony. Roy would grimace and moan, his voice vibrating with the rapid pulse of uncontrollable shaking. Sometimes these spasms were so intense they would throw him out of his chair, trembling on the ground, unable to pull his limp body up from the floor. These spasms also made his physical therapy painful and arduous, yet there was no avoiding the prescribed regimen. The muscles in his legs were weak from years of disuse. Had Roy not engaged in therapeutic exercises, which involved stretching and rotating the legs, his neuromuscular problems would have grown worse. He faced these tedious sessions with dread and loathing.

Roy had spent several years seeking relief from these torturous spasms. Many physicians prescribed a vast regimen of painkillers and muscle relaxers, but the heavily intoxicating and sedating side effects of these medications made Roy feel as if he were losing even more control over his own body. Alternative treatments like acupressure, acupuncture, meditation, massage therapy and aromatherapy offered little relief.

He finally decided to see a highly recommended pain specialist. I accompanied him on his first visit to the clinic. The doctor reviewed Roy's medical history and observed him carefully.

When he was finished, the doctor checked to make sure the examination room door was closed securely, then sat down with a somber expression on his face.

Speaking almost in a whisper, the specialist said, "Let me be frank with you, Roy. There is not a lot I can do for you and your pain will probably worsen over time. It appears that you have tried every legally available remedy." The doctor paused and sighed. "I'm not sure how you will feel about this, but we have accumulated quite a bit of anecdotal evidence that smoking marijuana can ease spasms and eliminate some of the pain, without the drastic side effects of those other pharmaceutical drugs. Unfortunately, I can't prescribe it for you. Technically, I can't even recommend it. My license could be suspended or revoked if I was caught talking to you about cannabis. The only reason I'm telling you this is that so many of my patients have claimed it is effective. If you have a way to obtain some marijuana, you may want to consider it as an option."

Several days later Roy called me at home, elated and excited. "Can you come over here right now? I have something to show you and you won't believe it unless you see for yourself!"

I hopped in my car and soon I arrived at Roy's apartment. When I walked in, I noticed a sweet aroma in the air, one I had not smelled since my teenage years. Roy lay in his bed, grinning. "This stuff really works! Here, grab hold of my leg and stretch it out."

I gently took Roy's wilted, atrophied leg in my hands and slowly straightened it. There were no spasms. Then I pushed his leg up towards his head and there were only minimal tremors in his toes. Normally, this type of movement would have racked his entire body with pain and spasms. My eyes widened. "This is amazing!"

Over the next several months Roy continued to smoke approximately two small joints each day and I witnessed the physical and emotional transformation of my friend. Since he was no longer continually awakened by spasms throughout the night, the black circles under his eyes disappeared. His appetite increased and he didn't skip meals anymore. He went outside at least once a day. He smiled and laughed frequently and his suicidal thoughts subsided.

The unfortunate price of Roy's relief was fear—the fear of being thrown in jail. Whenever he smoked, he completed an elaborate ritual of protection that involved pulling the curtains closed, tossing a towel over the gap at the bottom of his front door and spraying enormous amounts of air freshener.

While Roy lived in fear of the police, a few patients enduring excruciating pain like his had found a way to legally gain relief. One of the most vocal of these was George McMahon. I met George for the first time in 1998, when he spoke at the University of North Texas. He and his wife, Margaret, were traveling the country in a modest motor home, speaking to legislators, law enforcement officials, educators, health care professionals and anyone else who would open their ears and minds to the therapeutic value of marijuana for those enduring pain. I had the opportunity to spend several hours with George after his appearance at UNT, sharing our stories and hopes for the future.

I met George in his role as an activist, but I grew to know him as my best friend. He has been an inspiration to me. Here was a man who had fought and won the legal right to use cannabis, whose health was maintained by his government supply. He easily could have been complacent, enjoying the benefits of having secured consistent, regulated access to his medicine. Instead, he was fighting for the rights of other patients, speaking out day after day and investing a huge amount of his time and personal savings into educating people about medical benefits of marijuana.

George saw the quest for compassion and enlightenment as a personal mission and he told me that the opportunity to help others gave him the courage and strength to get up every morning. He struck me as a humble man, with a strength that belied his illness.

The day I first approached George about the prospects of writing his biography, I sat on a couch next to him in his living room while he smoked a joint. Neither of us had ever embarked on a project of this magnitude and self-doubt would prove to be our first hurdle.

George gazed at me skeptically and spoke in a gravelly voice that reminded me of asphalt, ashtrays and Iowa corn. "Do you think that people out there in the real world will be interested in reading a book about my life?"

"I think your story has tremendous value," I replied. "I believe it has the power to change lives."

"Maybe my story is worth telling, but I think the same thing is true about other people," he remarked. "Everyone has a story to tell. Most people just need somebody who knows how to tell it in a way that grabs people and pulls them in."

"As far as publishing, marketing, distributing and sales, I can't make any promises. Edgar Allen Poe wrote beautifully, but that didn't prevent him from dying a pauper," I cautioned.

George smiled. "I may not be a pauper, but I'm already a proletariat. Look at this place, for starters."

I glanced around the room and turned back to George. "Then what do you have to lose by trying?"

"You think you've got what it takes to craft a silk purse out of this old sow's ear?"

"You aren't a sow's ear and I promise to give you the best I've got."

George lifted his hand in the air and flexed his fingers. "I'm warning you, my bones are brittle and the joints in my fingers won't let me type long paragraphs. I'm going to need help."

I pulled a micro-cassette recorder out of my jacket pocket and placed it on the couch between us. "Not a problem, George. You just talk and leave the typing to me."

"It could be a long haul. You sure you're up to it?"

I paused for a moment to consider the potential ramifications of writing this book. I knew how difficult it would be to have a rational open dialogue with individuals who are adamant about their beliefs, especially in America, where the First Amendment is sometimes treated like so much worthless toilet paper.

I looked up at George and said, "I can take the heat. How about you? You have to listen to your own heart. Are you sure you want to write the book?"

George stared down at the coffee table as he put out his joint. After a deep breath, he turned to me and said, "Let's do it."

We began somewhat traditionally, with George pouring out a lifetime of memories into the tape recorder. The idea of encompassing the narrative inside a journey to Uncle Sam's marijuana garden grew naturally from the first tentative steps of the creative process and, before we were finished, the project had blossomed into a major road trip, documented by a video crew, including stops at the state capitol building in Little Rock, Elvis Presley's Graceland and the government pot garden at Ole Miss.

I believe the Compassionate IND program lies at the heart of a social and political conundrum that demands resolution. If the DEA, Supreme Court and federal legislators are correct in claiming that marijuana is a dangerously addictive drug with no medical benefit, then why has the government been giving it to sick and dying people for the last twenty-three years? On the other hand, if marijuana has medical applications, why is the federal government criminalizing patients, closing clinics and denying states the legal autonomy to resolve the issue independently? Assuming the Compassionate IND program was intended for research, then why have no longitudinal studies been conducted or reported by officials? It seems that the United States government is as confused about pot as is much of the society it represents.

However, the fact is that my friend, George McMahon, would not be alive today if it were not for his legal access to medical marijuana. Ultimately, the issue is not about laws, science or politics, but sick patients. Making no distinction between individual circumstances of use, the war on drugs has also become a war on suffering people. Legislators are not health care professionals and patients are not criminals, yet health and law become entwined in a needlessly cruel and sometimes deadly dance.

Truth is indeed stranger than fiction and this story proves it as well as any. The words you are about to read were transcribed from many hours of audio and video, drawn from days of conversation with George in ten different states over the period of a year. The book now stands as a human plea for compassion, an indictment of misguided and inhumane federal policies and a call for reform.

I sincerely hope our work will illuminate the irrational injustice of medical marijuana prohibition from the personal perspective of a man who had been suffering excruciating pain and walked "the green path," a man whose life was literally saved by legal access to cannabis.

Our journey down the green path has not yet ended...

— Christopher Largen

1

Insisto

Life is one big road with lots of signs
So when you're riding through the ruts
Don't complicate your mind '
Wake Up and Live Now
Wake Up and Live

– Bob Marley

Today is a good day. Every morning I say this to myself. Not a good day to die, like the Native American saying goes, but a good day to live. I was born with Nail Patella Syndrome, a rare genetic condition involving nail and skeletal deformities (among many other anomalies) that occurs in approximately 2.2 out of every 100,000 people. The signs and symptoms are quite broad and varied, but the most common ones are: an absence or under-development of fingernails or toenails; the absence or underdevelopment of kneecaps; malformation of bones, muscles and ligaments causing frequent dislocations; deformities of the elbows reducing mobility and rotation of arms and wrists; twisted legs and club feet; scoliosis or lordosis; kidney problems, in a few cases resulting in renal failure; and a higher rate of glaucoma. I know I might not have a great deal of time left, but I refuse to succumb without a struggle. Let death come sniffing and whining at my door like a hellhound in a cage, and I'll look the ugly beast in the face and scream, "Carpe diem!"

I've had more than my share of close calls. I rub the sleep from my eyes and gaze in my bedroom mirror, surveying the virtual road map of scars all over my body, most from major surgeries, some from fixing cars and digging ditches. The scars on my hands and legs are barely visible, but the dark one that twists and turns, stretching all the way down and across my torso, looks like the Mississippi River flowing into the Gulf of Mexico.

I fish through my bureau for something to wear. Most of my clothing has the obligatory rips and stains of a blue-collar background. Until I became disabled, I was proud to handle dirt, heat and metal. In rural Iowa where I come from, I wore a patch on my jeans like a badge of honor and I worked on cars, airplanes, houses and farm equipment.

Although I owned my own business and I was intellectually capable of administrative or clerical employment, I didn't want to shuffle paperwork, crunch numbers or sell people a bunch of stuff they didn't need. Even when my body was falling apart, I thrived on making things work. I simply never would have been suitable for a corporate office job.

Not that I won't wear a suit. When I speak before large groups of people, I usually don my blue pinstripe and my Tom and Jerry tie. A suit communicates respect and in turn it commands respect. Besides, I don't want my audience to pigeonhole me as an aging hippie pothead or a radical activist, two stereotypes that don't accurately reflect who I am. I'm just a normal guy and I don't like to generalize or be generalized.

Last night I packed my coats and ties for a road trip, but I won't need them until I climb the steps of the Arkansas legislature. This morning I want to feel comfortable. I need something I can breathe in. I grab one of my favorite shirts with a pattern that looks like a field of cannabis leaves and a pair of blue jeans.

My wife Margaret has awakened early to prepare for our journey and the scent of percolating coffee drifts into my nostrils while I throw on my clothes. I take mine black, no cream or sugar to mask the taste. Kind of like my life.

Margaret meets me in the hallway and hands me a warm mug of steaming caffeine. "Here you go, George." She doesn't ask me how I'm doing. She's been with me long enough to know that mornings are usually quiet for me until I've smoked my first joint.

I don't know what I would do without my wife. We've been to hell and back for over thirty-one years and she has pulled me back from the brink of death on more than one occasion. Whether she's kissing my neck, licking my wounds or chewing me out, she sure keeps me going. In sickness and in health, as they say.

My children gaze at me from several hanging portraits on the hallway wall. Margaret and I have three children and seven beautiful grandchildren and they all like me in spite of the fact that I can be a royal pain in the neck. Even after all these years, I still find it amazing that I have so much beauty in my life.

I'm really proud of my kids. They filled my highest dreams for them, which was basically that they would all grow up to be good people. I hope I've helped to give them a better world to live in when I'm gone. The abiding love of my family is the measure of my success in life, and I'll take that with me to the grave.

I step into my office to check E-mail. My study is decorated with various keepsakes from my travels, like a United States flag woven from hemp fiber, which makes it historically authentic. Many people don't realize that the first American flag was woven with cloth made from hemp. The pioneer wagons were covered with hemp canvas as they made the arduous journey to the Pacific. Even the initial drafts of the Bill of Rights were scrawled on hemp paper.

Next to my hemp flag is a beautiful banner of vibrant green, yellow and red, with a giant cannabis leaf painted in the center of it. The material is adorned with the words: A SPLIFF A DAY KEEPS THE DOCTOR AWAY! I carry this with me when I speak at universities and most of the students think it's great. Some have even offered to buy it from me, but I only have one and I'm not parting with it.

I have several tomes on the bookshelf in my study, including works by Steinbeck and Shakespeare, several copies of *High Times*, books on medical cannabis and photo albums filled with snapshots from my cross-country travels and travails. Pressed between the pages of one of these scrapbooks is my illustrious Certificate of Heroism, decorated with ornamental calligraphy, and signed by former first lady and drug war hawk Nancy Reagan. It provides me a healthy dose of comic relief from time to time. I have often wondered if Nancy actually considered me a hero, or if she even knew what in the world she was signing.

It doesn't really matter. It's all pomp and circumstance to me. I've got official paperwork that proclaims I'm a hero, but I sure don't think of myself that way. I'm just a person trying to get by in a chaotic world where drug lords, pharmaceutical executives and government officials get rich, while suffering patients trying to get relief go to jail and die.

I sometimes think of myself as a loner, because I don't identify myself with any groups. Politically, I'm independent and I try not to work with many activists if I can help it, even when it comes to medical marijuana. I've been burned too many times by people I thought were friends.

I'm not a Buddhist, a communist, a fundamentalist, an elitist, an evangelist, a Maoist, a Taoist or any other -*ist*. I'm a human being and I march to the pulsing, insistent beat of my own drummer.

Only one person has sent me an E-mail this morning. No form letters from politicians. No cyber-activists wanting to drain my wallet or advertisers looking to jerk my chain.

I scan all E-mail messages I receive for viruses, just to be safe. I'm not being paranoid. Some twisted people will go to any lengths to silence an idea whose time has come.

The one E-mail I received today is successfully scanned and I open a message from a desperate man...

I'm amazed by your story. I have cancer and arthritis that become more excruciating every day. The pain is so bad I can't sleep. My doctor is constantly increasing my painkiller dosage however, the medication weakens my immune system and I'm afraid the cancer will spread. If only I could get some relief, then maybe I could sleep through the night and be better able to cope with my illness. If there is anyone you think I can contact for help, please let me know.

People who are suffering often ask me if I can help them find medical marijuana. As much as I sympathize with their painful situation, I tell them that I can better assist them by continuing to be a legal cannabis smoker, a living testimony to the therapeutic benefits of marijuana and an advocate leading the fight for others suffering the way they are. If I violate the federal rules, I risk being thrown out of the program and I can't afford hundreds of dollars a month for black market medicine. Within a few months of not smoking, I could be in a critically terminal state.

I write the gentleman a short reply letting him know that I would be happy to provide him with any clinical, anecdotal or research information he needs, but I can't help him with actually obtaining marijuana.

It gets really tough at times to deal with all the letters from patients. On those rare occasions when I'm feeling too sick or tired to answer my mail for a few days, I have to postpone answering them, but eventually I answer each one. I would never just delete them.

I never asked to be in this position, but here I am and all I can do is try to teach people. It feels like an enormous responsibility and it keeps me awake on some sweaty, restless nights. But it's also the reason I pull myself out of bed in the morning

Today I glance over to the corner of my office where twenty large, silver canisters are stacked up four feet high. Each one is plastered with a prescription label from the federal government. They look like military ration containers, but they hold my medicine.

Once upon a time there were 6,000 joints in those cans, produced for a now defunct Food and Drug Administration program called Compassionate IND (Investigational New Drug). The program in which I take part was originally implemented in 1976, as the result of a lawsuit filed by a courageous glaucoma patient named Robert Randall. Marijuana helped him maintain his ocular pressure and, therefore, his sight. After being arrested for growing his own medical marijuana, he demanded the federal government recognize that smoking cannabis was a medical necessity for him. The federal officials compromised. They would acknowledge his medical necessity defense, but the government would be the sole supplier of his marijuana. Thus the Compassionate IND program was born.

Throughout the late nineteen seventies and eighties, there were only a few dozen applications to the IND program. The bureaucratic gauntlet of paperwork facing potential applicants was so daunting that most patients were unable to find doctors who were willing to deal with the nuances of a system bogged down in a minefield of minute details.

In the early nineties, spinal cord injury advocates and AIDS patients assembled a packet, available to doctors and patients, which both streamlined the bureaucratic paperwork and walked physicians step-by-step through the arduous process. This allowed many more applications to be submitted to the government.

By 1991, the federal authorities were staring at hundreds of applications from all over the nation. They knew they had to make a serious decision. They could grow more marijuana, supply it to patients and effectively admit that marijuana was medicine or they could shut down the program.

In 1992, under the Bush administration, the Compassionate IND was closed to all new applicants. The Secretary of Health and Human Services, Dr. Louis W. Sullivan, gave his direct order and the federal authorities flushed all those completed applications, along with the hopes of sick and dying people, down the proverbial septic tank. The patients who were already receiving the government marijuana, like myself, were grandfathered into the program. Theoretically, at least, we will receive marijuana from the government until the day we die. Nine of the fourteen patients have already succumbed; I am one of only seven remaining federally legal, marijuana smoking patients in the United States.

I can't speak for anyone else, but I'm not going quietly. I do have manners and I'm not screaming in anyone's face, but I am determined that the truth of my experience will be heard. Marijuana saved my life. Ten government joints a day have thus far given me twelve good years of living.

I grab my last full can of cannabis. The white storage label reads:

Marijuana Cigarettes
Approximately 300 cigarettes per can
Net Weight = 271.14 g
Average Weight per cigarette = .901g

Manufactured April, 1999
I.D. No: 9497-0499-103-4683
Research Triangle Institute

I pull off the lid, exposing a layer of Styrofoam designed to preserve the quality of the herb over a period of years. I peel it back and gaze down at 300 tightly packed joints, a month's supply, grown and distributed by Uncle Sam.

The marijuana is mid-grade cannabis sativa and it meets my needs, but I wish the officials would let me roll my own joints. That way I could use the right dosage size and roll them in much thinner papers without the thick glue resin the government uses. They do clean and process the raw marijuana. Of course, some dead seeds and stem materials survive the cleaning process, which I later have to clean out. I never manage to remove all the garbage, but I do get rid of most of it. This is no easy task, since my hands are deformed from repeated breaks and dislocations and my finger bones are brittle.

Uncle Sam freeze-dries my herb immediately after post-harvest drying, before they ship it to my doctor, in order to sterilize the seeds and preserve the potency of the leaf. It's an effective and efficient way to ensure that people aren't growing strains of government pot. That means I have to moisturize my medicine with water. Otherwise the leaves are simply too dry to smoke comfortably and it also wastes the medicine, because it burns too quickly for me to inhale what I need.

The researchers and scientists at NIDA do their best to deliver a high-quality product, even as they walk the precarious tightrope of government regulations. Compared to all the patients who live in fear of arrest and pay hundreds of dollars each month to get black market medicine of questionable quality, I have it easy. I just cut open the joints, clean out the seeds and stems, moisturize the herb and re-roll the joints with my own papers.

I'd probably try eating my marijuana occasionally if the federal government would allow me to, but it's prohibited under the rules of the program. No hash browns, no pot brownies and if certain officials at the Drug Enforcement Agency have their way, no hempseed nutrition bars either. And yet hemp seeds are quite nutritious. They contain protein, vitamin A, vitamin B, vitamin C, vitamin D, vitamin E, dietary fiber, calcium, iodine, iron, magnesium, phosphorus and zinc. A handful of seeds can provide the minimum daily protein requirement for adults.

Despite all the flak about the inherent dangers of smoke inhalation, the bureaucrats actually *require* me to fire up rather than chow down. Federal regulations stipulate that I can't smoke out of a pipe, either. Not even water pipes that cool the smoke and decrease the amount of tar. That's alright, because I tried water pipes and vaporizers and they don't work for me. The paperwork states that I must take my medicine in a paper tube and, of course, it must be government-grown cannabis, not black market weed.

Officials won't even let me use Marinol. That's fine with me, because I've never wanted to take it. Marinol (dronabinol) is a synthetic form of THC, just one of the many cannabinoids and other active substances found in the cannabis plant, the one believed to be the most psychoactive. Marinol has been approved for use as an antiemetic for chemotherapy-induced nausea and vomiting and in March 1993 it was also approved as an appetite stimulant for AIDS patients with the wasting syndrome. It is a Schedule III drug, which means it is legally available to treat a wide spectrum of symptoms, from headaches to eating disorders, but only by prescription.

Some patients have had positive experiences with Marinol, but people suffering from nausea or stomach cramps often can't keep the pills down. Additionally, Marinol can take hours to work and it leaves many patients feeling groggy and disoriented. Additionally, Marinol is very expensive. The pills can cost as much as seventeen dollars each. At three pills a day, it really stacks up. I'm not against the legal availability of Marinol to those who could benefit from it, but I think there should be several delivery systems available to meet the unique needs of individual patients.

In all the years I've smoked federal herb, I've never seen the acreage at the University of Mississippi where the government grows my cannabis. I'm not really sure that I want to see it. The thought of all that medicine locked up, while so many people are hurting, makes me angry.

From what I have heard, it's an outdoor growing operation, administered by bureaucrats and implemented by scientists. Friends have told me that two razor wire fences encage the pot plants, which are patrolled by drug dogs, monitored by motion detectors and guarded by armed security personnel with nighttime search lights. Sounds like a Fort Knox.

After the researchers and students in Mississippi harvest the marijuana crop, they ship it to Virginia, where it's processed, rolled and then stored in a locked freezer until my doctor orders it. Finally, they send it to a secure federal dispensary, where my doctor picks it up.

It's hard to believe, but I can walk into any pharmacy in the country and get drugs that have severe side effects, fatal overdose levels and can be addictive, but because I moved to Texas, I have to go across several states to Iowa once every four months to get my natural herbal medicine.

I grab several joints out of the packed canister, re-roll them and put them in a prescription bottle. I'm going to need them for the road and I take some extra papers, just in case.

I won't be taking this journey on my own today. Margaret will be at my side in the truck and she has agreed to handle the driving, all the way through Texas, Arkansas, Tennessee and Mississippi. She almost always handles the driving on trips. Long days of travel tend to wear my body down and to stop the pain, I smoke my medicine about once every hour and a half. I take proof of the legitimacy of my doing this with me. I don't want any trouble from an overzealous, misinformed police officer.

Although I avoid driving whenever possible, I'm well accustomed to travel and I exercise caution. I try not to drive at night and I don't take long trips by myself. Even though I am a legal smoker, I can still be cited for driving under the influence if my driving is significantly impaired, so I'm careful and act responsibly.

Some people fear that marijuana will significantly impair my coordination and alertness while driving, but the medical tests

have allayed those concerns. Moreover, if I get behind the wheel
without my medication, I'm prone to spasms, pain and nausea,
which are much more dangerous than the relatively mild side
effects of cannabis.

To spread the word of the therapeutic effects of cannabis
that have changed my life, Margaret and I have journeyed across
the world during the past decade, including Canada, Germany,
Holland and most of the states in America. In two years of criss-
crossing the United States, we literally ran the wheels off our
motor home.

It was absolutely worth every penny to help my fellow
patients, although one morning my wife and I woke up flat broke. At
that point, we were forced to take a temporary hiatus from traveling.
We settled in eastern Texas, amid sticky pine trees, pickup trucks and
pet dogs, in order to be close to my elderly mother who lives one
block from our home on a lake.

In my years of travel, I've come across the best and the worst
of humanity. I've talked with senators, professors, students, health
care professionals, police officers, patients and anyone else willing to
lend an ear. I tell them that throughout world history, cannabis has
been used as an herbal, symptomatic therapy for patients suffering
from gout, rheumatism, malaria, beri-beri, boils, chorea, constipation, diarrhea, dysentry, fever, insomnia, sexual dysfunctions, muscle
cramps, menstrual cramps, bladder spasms, muscle spasms, convul-
sions, headache, hysteria, neuralgia, sciatica, tetanus, hydrophobia,
ague, cholera, leprosy, rabies, coughs, fibromyalgia, cancer, AIDS, eye
strain, brain tumors, gastric ulcers, indigestion, dental pain, glaucoma, spinal cord injuries, brain fever, gonorrhea, hay fever, asthma,
bronchitis, catarrh, tuberculosis, piles, flatulence, dyspepsia, diabetes,
delirium tremens, impotence, depression, cardiac palpitations, ver-
tigo, sickle cell anemia and hepatitis-C, among other disorders and
illnesses. Although marijuana is not known to cure any disease or
injury, it does relieve associated symptoms and often assists in pre-
serving quality of life. I also tell people that I'm aware of the studies
and evidence, but I don't need statistics and research. I am living
proof that cannabis is good medicine.

I sip my coffee and look over the world atlas maps on my desk. Over the next four days, Margaret, Christopher and a three-person video documentary crew will journey eastward with me to the state capitol building in Little Rock, after which we will journey to Memphis to see Graceland before heading south for the federal pot farm on the distinguished campus of Ole Miss at Oxford, where researchers grow my marijuana.

Come to think of it, that's a lot of state lines to cross while carrying marijuana. It's a damned good thing I'm a federal patient. Otherwise, I would have to leave my medicine at home, which isn't an option for me.

In the past, I have run into serious trouble with international travel. When I went to Canada, the federal authorities had no problem with me bringing my marijuana into their country, but United States customs officials wouldn't let me return with my medicine, despite the fact that my medicine was grown here by the United States government.

I sit back in the wooden chair and light up my first joint of the morning. On average I'll go through ten marijuana cigarettes a day, which is what my protocol recommends. In addition to adjusting dosage by the number of joints smoked, it can be altered within limits by changing how much smoke is inhaled, the time between inhalations and the number of inhalations taken. For me, it all depends on how I'm feeling that day. On good days I smoke a little less, but when I'm hurting I need a bit more.

My friend Christopher comes shuffling into my study with puffy eyes, his long black hair in disarray. He clutches a Winnie-the Pooh pillow in one hand, to remind him of his son and daughter, and a mug of coffee in the other. He croaks, "Morning, George."

"Good morning. Was that sofa comfortable? Did you sleep okay?"

"I hardly slept at all. Too wired about the trip."

"You look like hell, man."

He chuckles and says, "Thanks, George. That really means something, coming from you."

He sits down and slurps his java. I think he ruins his coffee with the cream and hazelnut sweetener, but who am I to judge? To each his own, I say.

Christopher has been good to me over the years, one of those men who will step up to the plate when the chips are down. When I needed someone to drive with me to the federal dispensary in Iowa to pick up my herb, he was there by my side in a matter of hours. In a world where doublespeak is the norm and enemies often fight on the same side with you, he's a rare companion.

After I finish my joint, we walk into the living room and I grab my car keys off the top of the entertainment center. Contrary to the popular mythology about short-term memory loss being associated with marijuana use, I don't often forget where I put things. The landmark Missoula study results revealed that my memory is fairly dependable, even regarding some things I would rather forget.

Christopher and I step onto the front porch to watch the sunrise and survey my home one last time before we hit the concrete and white lines of rural Texas. I live in a quiet gated community that sits on a peaceful lake. The place is humble, but it's mine. I could walk away from it at any time, but I would also defend it with my life.

I look down to see the red clay bricks I've painstakingly placed, one by one, to form a small pathway from my front door to the edge of the yard. A few resilient blades of green grass push their way through spaces in between the bricks. It's taken Margaret and me several months to complete this path.

My wife also deals with major health problems; she contracted viral encephalitis in 1995. Aside from my fight to legalize marijuana for suffering patients, much of our remaining time and energy is spent taking care of each other. We don't have the strength and endurance to do much else, but we can still build a brick path together.

I wave to my next-door neighbor who has stepped onto her patio, still wearing house slippers, to let her dogs out for their morning romp. The people are friendly in this neck of the woods. They all know I use marijuana and many of them have seen me smoking on my front porch. Nobody judges me. Most of my neighbors live and let live.

I spent my youth in small mid-western towns, some of them sparsely populated by a few hundred people. Everyone there knew everybody else's business. I could always tell whether someone liked me or not. The ones who weren't fond of me might not strike up a conversation if they spotted me in a local diner, but they wouldn't hesitate to pick me up if I was stranded by the side of the road in a blinding snowstorm. There was an unspoken, yet seldom breached code of human decency in those rural areas.

My little mutt Barbie rubs against my legs, slapping my shins with her frantic tail. She can always sense when I am about to leave and it makes her nervous. I reach down to reassure her with a quick pat, but I can't fool her. Her doggy sixth sense is better than any truth serum and it tells her that I'll be leaving shortly.

Margaret steps out of our home and puts her arms around me. "Got everything?"

I have everything I ever dreamed of and more, I think. I've got a pretty good quality of life most of the time, loved ones who care about me, a dog that adores me and people who need me. I'm living on twelve years of borrowed time with no interest due.

"Yeah, Margaret. I've got everything."

A bluebird rhythmically chirps from the swaying branch of an oak tree in our front yard. His persistent call reverberates through the vast wooded area that surrounds my home. Our veteran motor home sits idle in the front yard, the bearer of many thousands of miles worth of tattered testimony to stubborn persistence or unbridled foolishness, you be the judge.

As I stand on the porch with my wife in my arms and my friend by my side, I wish I could somehow contain and preserve this moment before it passes into the murky waters of the past. I know that life is fleeting, however, and memory is fickle.

Christopher turns to me. "The tide waits for no man. Like we say, 'Patients are out of time.'"

He speaks the truth. I nod. At this very moment a man suffering with AIDS is feeling lonely and scared, because he isn't able to keep any food down and his immune system is failing. Somewhere a woman is hunched over a toilet while her young children listen to the retching sounds of chemotherapy-induced vomiting from behind the bathroom door. Right now a person with glaucoma is slowly going blind and wondering if he will see tomorrow's light. According to the federal laws of this free nation, sick patients who use marijuana to ease their pain are labeled common criminals. In the meantime, people are dying. And I am dedicated to bring their plight to the attention of those who could change it.

I pick up my small bag and follow Margaret to the truck. Like a hobo, I travel light, no extra baggage required. I get better gas mileage that way and the less I take the faster I move. Besides, I consider it a challenge to see just how many material possessions I can live without. I know that because of my illness, I could die on the road and it's not like I can bring it all with me anyway.

The bumper sticker on the back of my fiery red pickup reads: POLITICIANS ARE LIVING PROOF THAT SOME PEOPLE SHOULD EAT THEIR YOUNG. Christopher points to it and snickers. "I wonder what the Arkansas congressmen will think when they see that, George."

"I'll tell you, all the years of dealing with two-faced legislators and lying bureaucrats at the federal level hasn't done too much to restore my faith in the political process. Hopefully the congressmen won't take it too personally," I say with a wink.

Christopher has packed a huge bag of audiotapes for the trip. Even though I came of age during the sixties, I've never considered myself to be much of a fan of music. I usually prefer the delicate sound of a waterfall, the discordant cacophony of birds and wild animals or even the rumble and roar of a city street during rush hour. I want to hear the organic, gritty noises of real life. Not that I don't appreciate music. I still dig Elvy Musikka, John Prine, the Beach Boys, Miles Davis, Jimi Hendrix and many others.

Christopher has all of this and much more, including a lot of bands I've never heard of. He's got all kinds of music, from punk rock to classical. He once told me that he envied me because I saw Janis Joplin perform at the Filmore in San Francisco. I told him that my being there was a total fluke. I'd just happened to come along with some friends that night, trying to get out of the rain. I remember that Janis rocked back and forth onstage, gulping from a Jack Daniel's bottle, tearing out a little piece of her heart, bleeding for the people. I guess nobody could love her enough to keep her from killing herself.

As Margaret and I take off down the private road that leads away from our small plot of land, Christopher follows us in a green rental car, along with a documentary crew consisting of three students from the University of North Texas, ready to shoot on the fly. Their car is packed to the limit with video equipment, including three cameras, two tripods, a lighting kit, a computer and monitor, a television and a VCR. By ten o'clock this evening, I bet their Little Rock motel room will look like central command at the Drug Enforcement Administration.

I turn around and look out the rear window of my truck to see Christopher following closely behind Margaret and me, grinning like a Cheshire cat. I ease back in my seat for a moment wondering what the road ahead will bring. Then my mind revolves and I begin thinking of past roads which brought me to this point.

2

Bleached Beds and Hospital Halls

Sickness will surely take the mind
where minds can't usually go.
Come on the amazing journey
and learn all you should know.

— The Who, "Amazing Journey"

The blazing sun beats down without mercy on the vibrating hood of my truck as Margaret and I cruise down the rural Texas highway with Christopher and the documentary crew following in the green car. The humidity is unbearable. Over the years I have lived in many regions throughout the United States, though I'm still not sure which climates are easiest to bear.

On the one hand, a man can always throw on more clothes to protect himself from the freezing winter winds of Iowa, but there are only so many layers a man can strip off to relieve the sweaty fire of a southern heat wave. I swear I could be bare-ass naked and I would still feel like an egg frying in a skillet in the Texas heat.

The Gulf Coast air works its way into my bones, my muscles and my joints, causing me to feel that old familiar ache. Pain is like one of those family members you despise but grow accustomed to. I don't want any uninvited company today, so I reach over and grab my prescription bottle.

I received intensive medical care for most of my life and I faced life-threatening conditions on numerous occasions, due to kidney failure or medication reactions. My medical history includes nineteen major surgeries and the many specialized doctors who have treated me include urologists, neurologists, psychiatrists, osteopaths, orthopedic surgeons, general practitioners and chiropractors. I've been prescribed morphine, Demerol, Motrin, codeine, Valium and a multitude of anti-spasmodic, anti-inflammatory, tranquilizing, sedating and mood-altering medications. Over the years, I've swallowed a virtual rainbow of pharmaceutical antidotes.

This afternoon, however, I seek a simple, herbal remedy instead of a man-made concoction. As we wind our way through Texas highways, I twist the childproof lid off the brown bottle and pull out a marijuana cigarette, glancing up just in time to see a huge billboard advertising a popular pain medication that four out of five doctors strongly recommend. I swear it's enough to give me a headache.

I reach in my shirt pocket to remove the silver Zippo lighter Margaret bought me for an anniversary gift several years ago. Being sick and in pain for most of my life has taught me that very few material possessions have any lasting value. This lighter is one of those rare items, because it carries the indelible stamp of the woman who loves me. It's a simple treasure I carry with me on long journeys and it stays close to my heart in the pocket of my shirt.

I press the joint between my lips and light it, inhaling the sweet, fragrant smoke into my lungs. In a few minutes my pain has subsided, ebbing away like a pulsing ocean tide.

Margaret pops Roger Miller into the tape player and we listen to the king of the road sing, "You can't roller-skate in a buffalo herd, but you can be happy if you've a mind to." Happiness is indeed a state of mind, of being content with what is, rather than being angry with what can't be. I never thought there was anything I couldn't do if I set my heart and mind to it.

As Margaret drives, I continue smoking and memories of darker times in my life wash over me. It was long ago that my daily existence teetered unpredictably on a razor edge between life and death, but the memories remain close…

Illness cast a shadow over my earliest days like a constant, dreary companion I could not evade. From the moment of birth, I had mild deformities including missing fingernails, double-jointed fingers, poorly jointed elbows, a curved spine, a tilted pelvis and small kneecaps. Though nobody realized it at the time, these abnormalities were the result of a rare genetic condition that would remain undiagnosed for thirty-eight years.

At the age of three, I became intimately acquainted with the torturous nature of illness. Some scientists and philosophers might argue that disease is not evil, that nature wields an impartial sword, cuts deep and maims without preference or reprieve, but I learned that some disorders are so horribly excruciating that they can drive a man to do anything to stop the pain. It was a tough lesson.

In this particular instance, it involved my father, who was diagnosed with terminal tuberculosis. The symptoms, chronic illness and poor quality of life associated with advanced tuberculosis were unbearable to my dad and he feared the agony of a prolonged death. Once my father could no longer stand the pain of living with only half of one lung, he came home and grabbed my sister and me by the hands and started walking for the basement door. As the three of us marched through the kitchen, my mother and our next-door neighbor, sensing something was wrong, ran in behind us and snatched up my sister and me.

Despite losing his grip on his children's hands, my dad continued, as if nothing had happened, at the same steady pace through the door and down the basement steps. This was the last time I saw him alive. Within moments we heard two gunshots. My father had turned a rifle on himself. By embracing the executioner, he cheated the inquisitor. My family was left behind to pick up the shattered, bloodstained remnants of our lives. It was a tough lesson for all of us.

As I grew into childhood, my arms didn't develop normally. I lifted weights to compensate. Although this substantially increased my muscular strength, it also allowed me to pick up far more weight than my skeletal system could handle. I'd often break my bones while performing common daily tasks. These fractures occurred all over my body, but most frequently in my hands and wrists.

I was constantly falling seriously ill, more so than any of the other neighborhood children my age. During one prolonged siege of childhood illness, I contracted pink eye, followed by chicken pox, which then developed into strep throat and eventually ended with a major bout of rheumatic fever. I required six full months of hospitalization and an additional three months of bed rest before I could do any household chores or play the games that were typical for a normal boy of my age.

I couldn't believe it. I was nine years old and I could no longer swim, ride a bike or go fishing as I had done before. My heart experienced the typical yearnings of childhood daydreams, including thoughts of running barefoot through wildflower fields, but my body simply refused to cooperate. It seemed that my entire youth was shaped by the oppressive experience of being ill and it was a struggle not to be bitter.

Though I did not want to accept it, I slowly began to understand that I was fundamentally different from other children. I struggled with this idea for many years, taking a mental inventory of curious events in my life. For example, there were occasions when I could hit a brick wall with the full force of my fist, and nothing would happen to me or I'd merely skin my knuckles. Then there were times when I would simply pick up an object and my finger would break. I finally began to think, *No way, everybody is not like this. I don't know what is wrong with me, but this can't be normal.*

As a naïve child, I didn't realize right away that all people are "normal," each in unique ways, according to their own genetic codes and environmental histories. When it comes to the field of medicine, terms like "normal" are not accurate or descriptive and in some cases may actually be counterproductive since they pigeonhole patients, many of whom are already feeling alienated due to their disease or disability. Normality, like beauty, is in the eye of the beholder.

Nevertheless, many individuals definitely noticed that I was unusual and treated me differently because of it. For example, there have been occasions when others have insisted on helping me, without my asking, to complete relatively simple tasks, like hammering a nail. Perhaps they did it because they'd seen me fracture my finger doing something similar. Whatever the reason, I began to notice that somebody always stepped in to help me, whether or not I asked for assistance.

When I became aware that people were treating me differently, I began to wonder why. I thought that everybody had physical problems and pain and I didn't want anybody to think that I was incapable of doing the same activities everyone else did, so I simply didn't speak about it. I believed that bearing the burden in silence would somehow help me avoid the problem.

One winter, during my bout with rheumatic fever, I was yanked out of elementary school in the middle of the fifth grade and placed in a hospital. From my isolated room, in the dead of winter, I witnessed what I later thought of as a personal message, an omen from the wild side of nature.

I had risen early one morning, way before the sun came up, because I had been tossing and turning all night, soaking my sheets with cold sweat. My nurses and my parents had instructed me to stay in bed, but I stubbornly crawled over the bed rails and walked to the large window that was my sole connection to the outside world.

The somber sky was many shades of deep gray and the ground was spotted with the remnants of a soft blanket of fresh white Iowa snow. Although it was still quite dark outside, the snow was so bright that it hurt my tired eyes to look at it for very long.

I was about to turn away when I suddenly saw something moving at the edge of the woods bordering the hospital grounds. After a short time, a timber wolf emerged into a pasture, kicking up little chunks of dirty snow with his paws. I saw him for maybe ten or twenty seconds, just enough time to watch this tattered beast run across the field, only to disappear into his familiar womb of the woods. He never even paused to look at me. I remember thinking that the wolf was probably separated from his kin and I could relate with his solitary struggle for survival.

Soon after that incident, while I was still in the hospital, I read in the newspaper that a local farmer had shot and killed the last remaining timber wolf in Iowa.

It's one thing to be alone and quite another to be lonely. I felt a profound sense of isolation as I lay in my cramped hospital bed, trying to pass the days and nights. My bed rails were like the bars of a prison cell and I often felt like I was incarcerated inside my own body. Illness is a cruel warden.

Sometimes I was blessed with the company of a fellow patient, a child who had gangrene of the spinal column. We shared misery and laughs. However, with both of us being so sick, our contact with each other was sporadic throughout my treatments and his surgeries and the hospital staff wouldn't allow us to spend much time together.

Hours pass slowly for a young child in a sterile hospital room. After several weeks, time lost all meaning to me, but the incessant ticking of the clock on the wall reminded me of the water dripping from the icicles hanging from the eaves above my window and the distant promise of spring.

Once I returned home, the love and support of other people were vital to my sense of recovery and health. My loved ones helped me to regain a crucial knowledge of my place in the world after such a long absence. All visitors were welcome and everyone from my grandmother to our neighbors stopped by to see me.

Throughout my rehabilitation, my mother was engaged with work and parental responsibilities. As a widow, she was prepared to do whatever it took to ensure the survival of our family. She took her local beauty shop out of our home, moving her business to an uptown building. It was a good financial decision for the family and it freed up a room downstairs which was converted into my bedroom.

I was grateful for her compassion. My new bedroom had wide French doors that swung tightly closed for privacy, but could be opened when I wanted to watch the television in the living room from my bed. My screen companions were Lucille Ball, Bozo the Clown, Bart's Clubhouse, Playhouse Theatre, Jackie Gleason, the Lone Ranger and Roy Rogers, just to name a few. This newfound ability to instantly choose between solitude and community helped me recover more rapidly than I otherwise would have.

My close buddies would stop by frequently, including one friend who, due to a respiratory disease, had been stuck in an iron lung for an entire year. We were already accustomed to the idea of spending time together while one of us was sick, so my current situation didn't seem strange to us at all. Illness was simply another part of life.

I tried not to feel sorry for myself or dwell on the unfairness of my situation. I honestly thought that everybody adjusted to pain in some form or fashion. It was simply a part of existence. Trying to deny the pain hurt more than the pain itself, so I learned to live with it.

Between 1966 and 1968, I suffered from hepatitis, strains A and B. It was the "Summer of Love," but I was far from Woodstock. While the hippies and yippies had love-ins and swallowed magic mushrooms, peyote buttons and LSD, I lay in the hospital, getting treated with a variety of powerful painkillers, tranquilizers, narcotics, sedatives and anti-inflammatory drugs.

A few years later in 1972, finally recovered from the hepatitis, I wrecked my 1965, 150cc Honda Dream motorcycle. I was driving down a dark road one night, while under the influence of Seconal, a potent prescription sedative, and I misjudged a street corner, flipping and spinning through the air. The cycle hit me squarely in the face, pinned my head between the bike and the curb and cracked my helmet, but only after it dislocated my right knee and twisted my foot backwards.

I stood up and tried to walk. As I took a step forward, I noticed that my right leg was six inches shorter than my left, and my foot dangled backwards above the ground. I immediately fell to the warm pavement in excruciating pain, too dazed to think about anything besides mercy. I was in a state of shock, but not unconscious.

The ambulance arrived a few minutes later. One of the medical attendants, who told me that he had served as an emergency medic in Vietnam, reached down and felt my injured right leg, while a police officer shined a bright flashlight in my face. Then the ambulance attendant stared into my dazed eyes and spoke calmly. "Look, nothing is broke. We can fix this right here, right now. If I do it, it won't cost you anything. If you wait until you get to the hospital, it's going to cost you thousands of dollars. I'll need your permission and help to do it, but I believe I can pull your leg back into place right now."

I was dizzy from the medication and still in shock, but I absently said, "Sure, okay."

I heard the attendant say, "Sit on him."

Before I could protest, I felt my arms being pulled over my head. I immediately became alert as two cops, a paramedic and a bystander sat down on top of me. I could barely breathe as the attendant reached down, firmly grabbed my foot and twisted my leg and foot 180 degrees, turning the knee back into its socket.

There was no longer any influence of Seconal upon my brain. My mind was ruthlessly clear, my perception unbearably sharp. To hell with biker machismo, I thought, screaming like a baby with a diaper full of crap. After writhing on the ground for a few minutes, I somehow pulled myself up and walked with assistance.

Although the pain from the injury temporarily subsided, in time it became more intense. About three years later, my leg hurt so much it impaired my ability to function in daily life. At the time, I worked at the Kennicot copper mines as a laborer and plant operator, so I went to a company doctor. I was then referred to a specialist in Phoenix, who prescribed surgery to move the tendons in my leg that held my kneecap in place. When the specialist opened me up, he decided to realign my leg. He never told me he was going to do it and this really surprised me when I awoke and realized the doctor had reversed the inward step of my foot to an outward step.

To make matters worse, he put my cast on poorly. I reentered consciousness, screaming in pain, with this plaster cast crimped down on my leg. There were tubes running into the cast to catch and divert the fluids, but they weren't working properly, and the plaster was soaked with blood. I lay there for three days while the cast slowly filled with my life fluids, one painful drop at a time. The cast restricted the circulation in my leg, and my toes turned ice cold from the lack of blood.

I pleaded with a nurse to take off my cast, but the doctor refused to order the removal. The nurse finally told the physician, "I'm going to do it. I don't care whether you order it or not. His toes are turning purple!" After she stripped the cast, my leg became terribly swollen, which was just what the doctor was trying to avoid. There was no way they could recast it now.

It was several months before I could walk again. Even though I was in major pain, I refused to stay down. One day I rose up from my hospital bed and carefully shuffled to the toilet while biting my lip and groaning to deal with the pain. As I sat down on the commode, I felt a vague sense of accomplishment at completing this small task. Then I realized that I couldn't get back up off the toilet. I was forced to call the nurses to help get me out of the bathroom.

Being dependent on the assistance of others with a personal necessity like using the toilet was probably the single most humiliating aspect of being ill. I have always believed that a man should have privacy on his throne. I'd sit on the toilet for hours, closed off from the outside world, just to avoid having to rely on nurses rushing in to lift me off the john. One time I was absolutely determined not to accept any help, so I grabbed hold of the handicap rail and hoisted myself up to return to my hospital bed. I was so weak that I passed out, crumpled on the bathroom floor.

I was finally able to leave the hospital, although my right leg is permanently out of alignment, a painful and pointless outcome of surgical malpractice. Since that surgery, if I'm not careful when I walk, I can easily fracture or dislocate my ankle or knee. I've watched my step ever since—especially around knife-wielding doctors.

After a year, my knee still caused me incredible discomfort, but I didn't give up. I just gritted my teeth and tried that much harder. I wanted to be like other people who weren't always ill. I believed that my constant pain was a result of working and playing too rough. I had no idea that my fundamental genetic structure was screwed up, that I would never be like seemingly healthy, "normal" people.

I noticed that the right side of my body seemed to be more prone to injury, as it had always suffered the broken bones. In 1976, while working in the copper mine, I broke my right wrist. The doctor who treated me taped my hand in a fist position. Though my clenched hand appeared defiant when I held it in the air, I was resigned to submitting to the wiles of my misguided practitioners. After all, I thought, the doctors obtained extensive formal education and government licensure. They must know the critical details of my complex anatomy better than I do.

After a single maddening year of having my hand held in a

fist, my doctor finally removed the tape and it was discovered that I'd completely lost the joint in my wrist. Surgeons attempted to repair the damage by removing a piece of bone from my hip and transplanting it in my wrist. They hoped to fuse the joint, but failed and my right wrist gives me problems to this day.

In the early eighties, long after I left mining, I bought an auto-body shop. The shop was a great source of revenue and, more importantly, pride. I had become an apprentice auto-body repairman back in 1968 and soon thereafter earned a trade-school degree in auto-body work. Although side-tracked by mining and other pursuits, I was thrilled to finally get into the line of work for which I had extensively trained. Despite being in constant pain, I truly enjoyed my work.

I was able to perform my job until 1983, when I fell off a ladder onto a concrete floor, causing extensive spinal damage. Already accustomed to moderate levels of pain, I ignored the severe discomfort until it became unbearable and I couldn't sit up or walk. Then I had no choice but to seek professional help.

I tried ultra-sound treatments, but these failed to provide any relief for my back, so in 1985 I went to a chiropractor for spinal adjustments. I got some relief for three days, but then I became terribly ill and I was rushed to a local hospital where I was given huge amounts of morphine. My condition was diagnosed as renal failure and my right kidney shut down.

The doctors were respectful, but vague with any information about my health. The nurses, on the other hand, gave me the information I needed. They looked in my eyes and told me that I was probably dying. They knew it was important for them to be honest and for me to understand what was happening.

On September 27, 1985, I was given an emergency transfer from the private hospital where I was being treated to the University of Iowa where urologists attempted to save my kidney. Following the lithotripsy (a procedure in which shock waves are used to break a kidney stone into tiny sand-like particles), nine surgeries and the passing of numerous huge pieces of tuberculous stone from my kidney, things began to improve, but I was rushed into surgery again when my kidney stopped functioning for the second time. During this surgery my swollen and hardened kidney hemorrhaged profusely. My kidney erupted, spattering a surgeon's face with blood, urine and hard pieces of stone.

I actually became alert during this particular surgery, despite the heavy use of anesthesia. There was an entire team of doctors in the operating room when I regained consciousness. Four assistants had their hands inside of my abdomen, trying to pull my thick torso muscles apart so the chief surgeon could access my kidney.

I found myself staring into the face of something much worse than death. I had always been skeptical about the whole theology of divine punishment and eternal condemnation. Up until the moment I opened my eyes on that hospital table, I thought the concept of hell was a fractured fairy tale for spiritual masochists. Yet when I awoke to feel myself being carved up like that, I could have sworn I was in hell.

Of course I was in absolutely incredible pain, but I was still alert enough to joke. The doctors gaped down at me in horror while they continued to stretch my side muscles open. I pleaded with them, laughing and crying at the same time. "I can feel that. You're really hurting me. I'll do anything. Man, if you'll quit doing that to me, I'll fix all your cars. I'll rewire your Jaguar. I'll rebuild your Cadillac and I'll even go get it. You just tell me where it is. I can borrow a trailer and go pick it up." I sure hope that was all I promised to do, because I don't remember everything I said.

One bizarre image from those brief moments of anesthetized consciousness during the surgery remains burned in my brain. I remember seeing an angel with a shining halo, hovering at my feet. It was difficult for me to interpret this vision. Could there have been a message in this apparition? Where was my mind? Did I have a religious revelation or was the appearance of this angel merely a fleeting, drug-induced moment of self-deluded profundity?

I wasn't willing to accept it as a sign from heaven. Though I was open to being proved wrong, I didn't hold much stock in supernatural events. It seemed like I was dreaming vividly with my eyes wide open. Perhaps something in my subconscious was telling me, "Life is good. You better seize it while you can." At the time I had no idea that I was coming out from under anesthesia in the middle of major surgery.

The doctors eventually abandoned the idea of getting their hands through my abdomen. Many years of hard physical labor had produced a virtually impenetrable mass of torso muscles that refused to yield to their persistent efforts. Their alternative solution was to cut directly through the muscle tissue itself. The incision almost sliced my mid-section in half, cutting me all the way from my navel to my spine on my right side. One of my major nerves was severed during this unthinkable invasion by sharp, sterile metal, resulting in tingling and numbness throughout my lower abdomen, groin and right leg.

Miraculously, my kidney suddenly started functioning again during the surgery. The physicians were relieved, but they still didn't know what to expect. They left my kidney intact but didn't close the opening, just in case my unstable condition warranted another procedure in the future. Everything went black for me as the doctors cleaned me up and rolled me out of the operating room.

I was carved and gutted, nearly a corpse.

I opened my eyes and heard the reassuring, tender voice of a female. Was it my guardian angel, a nurse or both? I tried to turn and see who was talking to me, but my entire body felt like it was burning.

I looked down at my torso and saw a mass of gaping, sliced, muscle tissue, slowly realizing it was my own. Four small steel rings, each about the circumferences of a BB, were barely holding the two halves of my right side together.

The calm female voice said, "Don't budge. I'm going to talk to you for a minute, George. You just lie there and listen to me talk to you, George. Lie perfectly still."

Her soothing words prevented me from trying to move and injuring myself even further. I quickly fell into a deep sleep, evading the pain for a few exquisite hours.

When I again regained consciousness my doctors were

there, standing at the foot of my hospital bed. One of the surgeons chuckled and said, "You've got to drive to Omaha and pick up my Cadillac convertible. You promised! You've got to haul it home and bring your own trailer!"

The doctors were glad to see I actually was still alive, but it had obviously been a horrifying experience for them. Western physicians are trained to deal with clinical applications in an emotionally detached manner. It's one thing to operate on a sedate, immobile organism, a quiet mass of tissue and organs. It's quite another to operate on a human being with open, pleading eyes, screaming in pain.

I learned that after witnessing my surgery, one of my physicians actually changed his educational emphasis from urology to anesthesiology, which meant an additional two years of schooling. He declared unequivocally that he never wanted to see a man become conscious during surgery again.

The doctors also told me that I had clinically expired for six minutes during the surgery. It suddenly dawned on me that my angelic hallucination was probably a near-death experience. I was only thirty-five years old, but I was already precariously poised at what seemed to be the final exit.

It has been said that pain is a great teacher. The most important thing pain taught me was that I didn't want to be in pain. It also taught me the true worth of the people who valued me even when I didn't have much to give.

During my prolonged recovery period there were very few visitors since I had no family in Iowa City and my wife was many miles away, struggling to make financial ends meet. This was fine with me. I didn't want many visitors, because I needed to remain focused on getting well.

The one regular visitor I had was a hospital employee named Steve White, a childhood friend who became a priest and later was diagnosed with severe schizophrenia. After that, he began working in the same hospital where he continued to receive cutting-edge treatment for his illness. He visited me three to four times a day like clockwork: a few minutes in the morning, for lunch at noon, a few minutes in the afternoon before he went back to work and often returning in the evening to wish me goodnight.

Although I enjoyed the company of my one frequent visitor, I made it clear to the nurses that I couldn't handle having other patients stay in the room with me. The hospital staff tried to give me a roommate once, but the man talked too much and he snored incessantly. I didn't want such an intrusive distraction from my therapy and healing and found him so annoying that his mere presence bothered me. If he moved his foot under his sheet, it was enough to make me scream. I was in excruciating pain. The last thing I needed was another complaining, noisy, sick person sharing my room. Once I made it clear to the hospital staff that I needed my privacy, the man was moved to another room and I was left blissfully alone.

The hospital staff adjusted to the fact that I preferred solitude. They kept my door closed all day long, leaving me alone with the soothing, buzzing hum of the florescent lights. They came to realize I needed the door shut to preserve my personal space for building back strength.

In order to pass the long hours of isolation, I began to re-read Hermann Hesse's monumental work, *Siddhartha*, a book that would forever change the way I dealt with pain. The story chronicles the life and spiritual journey of a young man whose search for truth and meaning leads him down the false paths of asceticism and hedonism, only to realize that true serenity resides in flowing, like a river, with the gentle rhythms of nature.

From the confines of my hospital bed, I began to practice contemplative meditation in order to quiet my anxious mind. I discovered that I could control my sense of pain by simply focusing on breathing in and out, in and out.

I started by counting my breaths and calibrating the lengths of my inhalations and exhalations. With time and practice, I no longer needed to control my breaths. I could succumb to the natural process of breathing and become one with my breath, so to speak. Rather than fight the pain, I was able to merely acknowledge the sensation, without judgment, and allow it to pass through me with my exhalation. This discipline eased my pain, helped me relax, lifted my spirits and assisted in my recovery.

Although I spent most of my time in solitude, I did develop a distinctly fraternal bond with the dedicated team of nurses and doctors who entered my room at intervals during my extended recovery. On many occasions I was asleep when they arrived, suffering from high fevers and night sweats. They would simply enter, look at my charts, observe me for a few minutes and then leave. At other times they would joke with me and offer their moral support. It was exactly the amount of camaraderie and friendship I needed. I just wanted people showing up from time to time as my friends, to lend me their courage and strength.

Three years after my release from that hospital, I returned to visit the nurses and physicians. Even after a prolonged absence, those dedicated professionals recognized me, throwing their arms open, giving me big hugs and saying, "You made it, man! We knew you could do it!"

When I had originally arrived at Iowa City Hospital, prior to my major kidney surgery, I was wearing a pair of worn-out overalls so dirty and stiff from hours of manual labor they could have walked on their own. After the surgery I had no shirt, no pants, and no socks. My wardrobe consisted of a green hospital gown that exposed my naked ass to the world. I didn't mind too much. After all, it wasn't like I was going to be ballroom dancing anytime in the near future.

As I got better, I was able to get around the hospital a bit. One day, I became acquainted with the parents of a young male patient who had just died in a room down the hallway from my room. They were naturally distraught over the untimely death of their son and they shared their deep sense of grief with me before they left the hospital.

The next day a nurse appeared in my room, holding socks, shoes, a pair of pants, and a shirt. She said, "A man and woman dropped these clothes off at the nurses' station and asked me to give them to you."

I knew right away the clothes belonged to the dead son,

who was similar to me in build and height. I was quite shocked by this simple gesture of generosity. What had I done to deserve this honor? I considered it for a moment, then slowly shook my head and replied, "Nah...I don't think so. I don't want any pity."

The nurse smiled. "It's not really about pity. Maybe you are going to have a chance to go on. You might need them. The parents hoped this would help you and I hope so too." She dropped the clothes on my nightstand and left the room before I could protest.

I was absolutely amazed. Almost all of the nurses acted like they were my sisters. They didn't complain about their sore feet and they never chastised me for ringing their buzzer too often. If they were humbled by my predicament, I was humbled by their compassion. Their warm glances and cheerful smiles nurtured my spirit and their kindness brought light and life to my bleak existence.

Nurses and caregivers are so wonderful to do what they do. I don't want to say it's a completely thankless job, but it can be extremely challenging because of the emotional attachment and potential loss involved. They must have loving hearts to devote their lives to taking care of patients, especially old crabapples like myself. I've been fortunate to have that level of compassion from most of the nurses with whom I've had contact.

Not all of the health care workers were supportive, however. One nurse snatched my pills away from me while I was convalescing. I'd been taking Demerol and Percodan for pain management and she tried to give me codeine instead. She thrust the pills into my hand and ordered me to swallow them.

I said, "I can't take those. They make me puke and I sure don't want to vomit in this condition. If I start retching, I could tear my side open."

She replied, "Oh, don't be silly. You can take them. The doctor ordered it."

I obediently swallowed them and, just as I predicted, they made me violently sick. I reported the nurse's actions to the hospital staff. She tried to deny the facts, but she was eventually transferred to another wing.

I'd created a confirmed enemy. To this very day when I visit that hospital, she glares at me with daggers of ice in her eyes and I return her bitter gaze with an amused, knowing smile.

During my hospital stay I participated in numerous research projects for medical departments including pain, urology, cancer, genetics and atomic medicine. I underwent CAT scans, magnetic resonance imaging and several rounds of tissue analysis. One time they put me up against a machine that was so complex, I can't even remember what they called it. The intimidating structure looked like huge bass drums from a marching band. It was some type of nuclear or atomic device that took pictures of my body at the cellular level. They graphed my anatomical system like an aerial road map.

At that point, I still didn't know if I was going to live or die, but I figured that regardless, this was one way I could contribute to a significant body of knowledge that would live beyond me and help other people. My participation also had the added benefit of giving me access to a plethora of physicians and specialists, each with their own perspectives on my condition.

An added traumatic experience during my recovery period was that the gaping surgical wound in my side didn't heal properly and soon became infected. The opening then had to be cleaned six times each day and the condition persisted for months.

When I eventually was discharged from the hospital, the doctors gave my wife a medical tool to take home with her to clean my wound. It looked like a turkey-basting instrument with a ten-inch catheter hose, designed to insert through a deep hole in my side about a third of an inch wide. It was a modern torture device, but it was going to save my life.

Margaret stared at the round hole in my flesh, her lips pressed together tightly. She held her breath with intense concentration, then carefully pushed the long tube through my muscle tissue and internal organs. Then she injected a dose of hydrogen peroxide directly into my kidney to control the unexplained infection.

My wife went through this brutal ritual every day, six times a day. This tested her commitment and endurance, but Margaret is a strong woman. When she sets her mind to something, as she did then, she is able to do most anything.

Over the following weeks, however, it became clear that Margaret could not handle administering these cleanings without some support. The treatment schedule was wearing her down. She demonstrated the horrible sterilization procedure for our children, so they could assist me when she was not around. Sometimes when Margaret and our children were away from the house, my friends were called upon to perform the task.

While I focused on getting well, my wife and children generously gave me their patience, tenacity and encouragement. I know it had to be one of the most trying times of their lives, but in our family there are no debts beyond forgiveness. I would have died a broken man had it not been for their support and I've found no greater love in life.

After seven months of constant battling with the unhealed surgery wound, my doctors discovered I had systemic tuberculosis, the disease that had indirectly killed my father when I was three years old. Tuberculosis had effectively robbed me of the man who gave me life. Now, the same disease was attacking me.

I was immediately placed on an intense anti-tuberculosis therapy program. One outcome of the treatment was that it aided my surgical wounds in healing. However, my surgical trauma wasn't over yet. Doctors performed one final surgery to remove four inches of decayed muscle and flesh that had built up around the area of the wound that hadn't been healing properly. Ever since, I carry a scar that looks like the Mississippi River meeting the Gulf of Mexico—twelve inches long, three-quarters of an inch wide, running into a four inch deep, six inch round hole, culminating inches from my spine.

The financial strains on my family were great and it was clear I would not be able to work anytime in the near future so, after filing mounds of detailed paperwork and hiring an attorney that specialized in the social security system, I was formally declared disabled late in 1987. I began drawing a monthly check from the federal government. This was difficult for me to fully accept, but I had no other choice.

I was raised in rural areas where many folks have a work

ethic that borders on being devoutly religious. I always valued my independence and I never wanted to rely on other people to take care of me. Although I wished I could continue to work, I was forced to begrudgingly face the fact that physical labor was no longer healthy or possible for me. It became clear that the next hole I dug could be my own, so I swallowed my pride and cashed the check.

I continued to travel to Iowa City, sometimes as often as two and three times a week, for ongoing treatment, observation and evaluation. My doctors were committed to finding the source of all my problems, but they remained completely baffled by my symptoms. I was repeatedly shuffled from one department and specialist to another, each working both independently and as members of an interdisciplinary team.

I felt like I was frozen in the middle of some absurd cosmic joke, but I wasn't laughing. It was as if every door I opened only led to another closed door. It was a struggle to find an existential sense of meaning and purpose in a journey that seemed to lead nowhere.

Finally there was a breakthrough when doctors diagnosed my condition as Nail Patella Syndrome (NPS), a rare genetic disorder. Although it is poorly understood, NPS is thought to affect major organs including the kidney and liver. It disrupts the immune system in ways that are difficult to understand, causing the bones to be deformed, become brittle and break easily. In addition, NPS also affects the joints, limits mobility and causes chronic pain, muscle cramps and spasms.

The disease is incurable, progressive and, in most cases, terminal. Many NPS patients are affected with organ and immune system complications, as well as other serious problems. In these cases, patients usually die from the disease before they reach the age of forty. Only a few hundred people have been diagnosed with NPS in medical history.

After all those years of waiting and searching, I finally had a concrete diagnosis. Even though the prognosis might be terminal, I tried to view the information in a positive light. At least now I didn't have to fear the unknown anymore. At least I knew the name of what might kill me.

Finally, I understood why I had been so sick throughout my life and why spells of nausea, fever, chills and night sweats were common occurrences. Now I knew why I got tired so easily and could only stand for a few minutes without experiencing unbearable pain. I knew why the muscles in my back and legs became constricted, causing intense pain. I understood why I had lost all my adult teeth by the time I was twenty-one years old (many NPS patients lose their teeth when they are very young). Being given a diagnosis and learning about the disorder from which I suffered was like fitting together the pieces of a jigsaw puzzle. Now I could connect the pieces of my life into a whole picture that finally made some sense.

Although I no longer felt like an alien, my mind was racing. I thought, *Goddamn it, I don't want to die. I want to see my kids grow up!* I was still very preoccupied with minute-to-minute survival while I was undergoing treatment, but I was driven by the knowledge that my wife and children needed me and this encouraged me to fight harder.

Nail Patella Syndrome would eventually impact my entire family. We discovered that my mother also has NPS, although she is only affected by slight joint deformities and glaucoma. Later in life, my older sister died at the relatively young age of forty-four from complications caused by NPS. After years of taking pharmaceutical drugs to treat a multitude of symptoms, her fragile system finally failed. My sister's death left me contemplating the absurdity and cruel randomness of disease and death.

I have mixed emotions regarding my tumultuous course of treatment prior to my diagnosis of Nail Patella Syndrome. After the diagnosis, most physicians treated me like a clinical specimen. I understand their interest as it is a very rare disease. Furthermore, in addition to the more common symptoms, there are some very unusual anomalies that are associated with Nail Patella Syndrome including digestive disorders, toxemia of pregnancy, abnormal pigmentation of the iris, attention deficit disorder, thyroid disorders, recurrent urinary tract disorders, poor teeth with thin enamel, spina bifida, cleft lip and cataracts. Nevertheless, I didn't like always being put under the microscope, especially by doctors with whom I developed personal relationships.

I feel a pronounced sense of anger at all those earlier practitioners who took advantage of me as a "lab rat," operating on me, pumping me full of prescription drugs despite not really knowing what was wrong and never taking the time to look at my symptoms as a part of a whole complex problem. They could have simply told me, "There's something different about you and you should go find out what it is." Instead they tried to fix each individual illness or injury, one band-aid at a time, but their seemingly altruistic attempts were hopelessly futile. So now I have the scars and results of unnecessary surgeries all over my body, a physical testament to the lasting wounds of misguided medical care.

In all fairness, I also had surgeries and treatments when I desperately needed them. I'm grateful for those committed, caring doctors who saved my life. They respected me enough to treat me like a human being. Nevertheless, I cannot help but harbor a residual distrust of the medical establishment, especially those members who push pharmaceuticals, wield scalpels carelessly and regard the making of money as more important than the welfare of patients.

I've spent an enormous amount of my early life in sick beds and hospital rooms. These rooms became embedded within my conscious memories like bleached nails in white walls, possessing both the comforting familiarity of home and the horrifying finality of a tomb filled with antiseptic odors and agonizing screams. There were many times when I wondered if I would ever leave alive. I didn't know that I already possessed the key to a great secret that would totally transform the rest of my days.

3

Illicit Relief, Dubious Doobies

The whispering sigh, exhaling breath
the clenching pain, a moments rest.
Or not, time crawls, each pain extends
and time grows short where pain's no guest.

– John Markes

Christopher pulls over to a greasy truck stop to pump his car's tank full of unleaded gas. Margaret and I pull in behind him. I climb out of my truck and glance around.

I've always loved the look and feel of places like this one. I take it all in, the faint smells of burning diesel and cow manure, the piercing call of a shiny crow perched on a rusted trashcan, the black oil spots from cars and trucks that stopped here during their travels across the country and the gaze of complete strangers, people who are all on different paths, who are all watching their own clocks, who have just enough time to offer you friendly nods but not enough time to be truly concerned with your business. Where do they come from and where are they going? Are they really going anywhere?

I've always been able to find mystery and irony in that which is seemingly mundane. It's like dreaming awake. I know it's just another day, one more turning of the squeaky wheel, but for one moment I feel like I've just stepped into a painting. Then I walk over to Christopher.

He leans on the car and says, "You ever hear about kids using gasoline to get high? I've heard it can cause serious brain damage, not to mention cancer."

I nod my head. "I know it was common in rural areas when I was a kid and now they do it just about everywhere. Some of my friends tried it growing up, but I never did. I had better sense than that. Most of the country kids don't huff gas anymore though. They prefer to go out and pick some weed instead. I never quite understood the appeal of it. I always figured gasoline goes in the car, not in my brain."

Christopher pulls the gasoline nozzle out of the car's tank and says, "I guess the DEA agents haven't cracked down on petroleum products yet."

I raise my eyebrows and say, "Give them time, Christopher." He smiles and I wonder if he thinks I am joking.

I head for the bathroom while he pays for the gas. A clock ticks on the graffiti-covered wall above my head and the cramped room smells putrid, a combination of bleach and urine. It's a far cry from home.

As I stand in the filthy bathroom staring at the clock, I think about how differently I now view time. My days are borrowed; doctors tell me I should have been dead twelve years ago. I try not to think about my life beyond the next few weeks and I don't like making concrete plans. I'm never totally sure how I will feel from one day to the next. Today I am able to trek across the country; I might not be able to get out of bed tomorrow.

I look down into the commode to check the flow of urine. I always have some blood in my urine, but it's not always visible. Protein in the urine is inherent in people with Nail Patella Syndrome. However, due to surgical and pharmaceutical damage wrought on my kidneys and bladder, I sometimes have urine the color of tomato juice. After long periods of being in a car or times of prolonged movement or physical stress, my system is weakened and I am more prone to this problem. The bloody urine can last for up to two weeks straight when I'm at my most ill. I have to be careful not to become too weak and sick to fulfill my mission. I know my limits and I treat them with respect. I only go on trips that I feel are very important and worth the risk of having blood in my urine. Today the fluid looks clear, so I zip up my pants, wash my hands and head out of the lavatory.

I walk into the truck stop convenience store, grab a bottle of water and get in line at the checkout counter behind Christopher who is buying a bottle of ginseng tea for an energy boost. I gaze down below the counter at the open market of drugs for sale. I see long shelves of aspirin, painkillers, alcohol, sedatives, stimulants, caffeine, nicotine and diuretics. A package claiming to contain an aphrodisiac promises to make a man's penis harder and his erection last longer. Near it, a liquid herbal concoction in a tiny vial claims to improve memory. Below that a bikini clad woman adorns a bottle that promises to reduce the pounds and inches in a few short weeks.

It's a virtual pharmacopoeia, this crass blending of capitalism and drugs promising instant health, instant improvement, instant gratification. As long as you've got the cash, you can walk into a corner store and pick any remedy you want.

Any remedy but mine, that is.

Christopher and I go outside and climb back into our respective vehicles. As my wife pulls our truck back onto the road to continue our journey, I think again about the array of pills and concoctions for sale in the convenience store. My mind spins back to the days when my own medicine cabinet looked like a pharmacy...

I used to gulp pills like a candy addict munching gumdrops. It seemed my doctors had a pill for everything. Pills to wake up. Pills to sleep. Pills to relax muscles. Pills to relieve pain. Pills to fight infections. Pills to flush all the other pharmaceutical toxins out of my weakened system.

I found myself torn between two terrible choices: I could either endure the physical pain that was so intense it would consume most of my daily energy or I could swallow the drugs that reduced my pain but numbed my awareness, while I sped toward an early, bitter grave.

Throughout the first three decades of my life, I did exactly what I was instructed to do by my physicians. I trusted the doctors and the Food and Drug Administration to know what was best for me. After all, I reasoned, clinical practitioners were required to have years of intensive education and training in order to receive their licenses to prescribe government-approved medications, therefore they must know what they are doing.

I really wanted to believe in my doctors and my government and looked to them with hope. I thought to myself, *These doctors know my body better than I ever could. These drugs have been endowed with a seal of approval from the Food and Drug Administration. Surely government officials would not allow these drugs to be prescribed if they were potentially lethal!* I was incredibly naïve.

In retrospect, I still believe that most of my doctors meant well, but most of us know what the road to hell is paved with. Good intentions aside, the drugs some doctors prescribed for me nearly caused my death on more than one occasion.

In the early 1960s, I started smoking marijuana on an occasional basis. Although pot smoking by teenagers and young adults would later become more visible in the media, it was not widely used by my peers at the time. I was to discover that my responses to marijuana use were quite different than those of other people. Unlike other individuals who got intoxicated and giggly after smoking marijuana, I simply felt better. I was more alert, my pain was not as debilitating and it was easier for me to move around. The spasms I suffered, particularly in my legs, which prevented me from sleeping eased after smoking marijuana and my legs didn't dance around on their own all night. I enjoyed the relief pot gave me, so I continued to smoke.

At the time, I thought these effects were simply byproducts of the euphoria associated with smoking cannabis. I had no idea that marijuana was actually providing physical, now medically proven benefits. Like some others who smoked pot, I worried about my habit and about how much better it made me feel. I assumed I had a problem with drugs. Ironically, I wasn't all that concerned about the regimen of prescribed substances I was swallowing on a daily basis, because they were dispensed by people I trusted—my doctors.

Years later, I was shocked when I learned that some people lie to their doctors or forge prescriptions in order to get the same drugs I had been taking. I didn't understand this phenomenon.

Because of my illness, I could get all the prescription drugs I wanted (and plenty I didn't want), whenever I wanted and I never needed to lie. I'd simply explain my symptoms and the physicians would immediately respond with physical therapy and drugs.

As I slowly realized how powerful these medications are and how they altered my moods and made me deeply depressed, I became convinced that taking them made me a common drug addict. I began to feel that the only difference between me and the sweaty junkies vomiting in dark alleyways, the ones I'd seen in public service announcements, were that my prescriptions were written by my doctors.

Throughout the mid 1970s my hands were in bad physical shape. I was employed in the mines, handling caustic chemicals and working with heavy equipment. My hands became terribly swollen over time and they often felt like they were on fire.

I lived in Arizona at the time and I became acquainted with many Mexican people, ranging from middle-aged to elderly. Our kind landlady was a wise and wrinkled *curadero*, a native healer, who noticed the severe swelling in my fingers.

One day she beckoned me with wizened hands to follow her to the back room of her home. As I stepped into a giant walk-in pantry, she spoke in a brittle voice, tinged with ancient knowledge from the windswept desert. "I have something that will help you." She reached up to the top shelf and revealed a tincture comprised of marijuana buds soaked in cane alcohol.

I was skeptical since I had never heard of marijuana being used as a topical ointment. I asked her, "Are you sure this is going to work?"

"I can assure you that Mexican peasants have used this herbal remedy for centuries. The buds have to be soaked only in cane alcohol to be effective."

She gently spread the potion on my aching hands. The rubbing compound initially made my hands burn even more, but after a short period of time the sensation subsided and the swelling disappeared.

After that, I stopped by the old woman's home once or twice a day during the week and four to five times a day over the weekend for applications of the healing potion to my hands. After several weeks my hands had completely returned to normal and I regained the use of my fingers with far less joint pain than before. I never again experienced the intense redness, irritation and swelling.

This elderly woman seemed to have no idea that she could go to jail for using marijuana tinctures. I was grateful to my land-lady for her illicit assistance.

By 1975, I became more comfortable using marijuana as I felt that in small quantities, it eased my discomfort and symptoms better than any prescribed drugs or combination of drugs. I wasn't, however, certain about the physiological benefits of marijuana. I was still concerned that I might become just another hopeless drug addict.

Nevertheless, I wasn't secretive about my marijuana use; I told everybody about it. In those days, it wasn't considered a hor-rible thing. The government's "war on drugs" had only been declared in 1970 and the public outcry wasn't what it is today. In fact, a lot of people didn't consider pot smoking a big deal. When I told my doctors I smoked marijuana, they always gave me pills instead, telling me, "Take these, they're better for you." They believed that swallowing toxic pharmaceuticals was preferable to smoking cannabis.

I loathed the intense side effects I experienced from ingest-ing prescription drugs. The medications had little effect on my chronic pain and spasms, but they left me mentally and physically incapacitated. Sometimes I felt so doped up that I just couldn't function.

I wanted to be a dependable husband and father, but I just wasn't as strong as the potent prescription drugs I was taking. I felt like I was living in a plastic bubble, separated from the people I loved most. My children and wife stood vigil while I spent day after day anesthetized on the couch, staring off into space like a zombie while the television blared advertisements for beer and flu medicine.

Throughout the early and mid 1980s, I continued to follow medical advice by swallowing my FDA-approved pharmaceutical medications. It took me several years of gulping pills before I realized that I was slowly poisoning myself. By that time, I'd already been rushed to hospital emergency rooms on at least six occasions, suffering from severe and potentially lethal conditions such as hallucinations, respiratory malfunctions and renal failure, all induced by the pharmaceutical drugs.

It was clear the treatments and pills caused all kinds of physical and mental problems and they weren't managing my pain. While smoking marijuana I didn't endure all the intense side effects of potent prescription drugs. But I still couldn't get past the deeply ingrained idea that marijuana was a recreational drug of abusers and that I really shouldn't be using it.

My thinking changed when marijuana literally saved my life.

I was recovering from major kidney surgery, the operation in which the doctors cut me open from my navel to my spine. I was lying like a gutted fish in my hospital bed, trying to maintain my will to live.

The doctors kept giving me pharmaceutical substances for pain, spasms and infection. The constant onslaught of prescription drugs ultimately damaged the lining of my stomach, leaving me in a terribly nauseated state. This damage rendered me incapable of digesting solid food of any kind and the constant pain prevented me from obtaining any rest. My health was in a serious downward spiral.

The situation became even more critical. I had not eaten solid food in thirty days and I was hooked up to IVs for nutritional sustenance, water and drugs. I had not slept for six weeks. My eyes never closed and I even stopped blinking. My doctors were waiting for me to die. One afternoon, a doctor told me that I probably only had about five hours to live. He advised me to get my final affairs in order and contact my family members and loved ones.

I pleaded with the doctor. "I want to go home, please. I don't want to die here."

The doctor shook his head and said, "I hate to tell you this, George, but I don't think you will make it that long. If you try to leave this hospital, you will probably die on the way to your house. Even if you make it home, you will certainly die there."

I simply refused to believe him. This doctor would never venture to predict the year of his own death, yet he seemed absolutely convinced about the hour of mine. In my mind, the arrogant certainty of science could not ultimately eclipse the mysteries of life and death. This was not the first time a doctor had made such a pronouncement, so I ignored his arbitrary sentence of death, just as I had in the past.

I phoned my wife to proclaim to her my undying love. Then, instead of directing her to make emergency funeral preparations, I told her that I would be coming home as soon as I was physically able to drag my weary self out of the hospital bed.

That night, a generous healthcare worker quietly entered my hospital room in the early hours of the evening. "Hey George, you got a minute?"

"Maybe one or two. I haven't got long, though."

"I have a message for you. There's a terminally ill cancer patient in a room down the hall. The doctor's don't think he's going to pull through. Anyway, he noticed the tattoo on your arm and wanted to ask you something."

I managed to gather enough energy and strength to slowly lift my hand in the air, so the attendant could view the faded tattoo of the Zigzag man, the one from an advertisement for rolling papers, on my left forearm. I had purchased this tattoo one rowdy night in 1974, fourteen years earlier, on a complete whim. When I decided to get it my wife was by my side as they poked the ink-filled needle into my flesh. I didn't know it at the time, but that tattoo was about to serve me well. "You mean this one?"

"Yeah, George. That's the one."

"What about it?"

"Well, this patient thought…I suppose I'll just come right out and ask. Do you smoke pot?"

"I have from time to time."

He paused and said, "I'm not trying to pry or anything, but this cancer patient wants to know if you would trade him a cigarette for a joint."

I glanced over at the four unopened packs of cigarettes on my nightstand. "Sure, man. Lord knows I'm not smoking any cigarettes. Not enough energy. He can have every cigarette I've got. I'm probably dying anyway. As far as the joint goes, I'm in so much pain I'm willing to try anything to get some relief."

He said, "Thanks, but the other patient said just one cigarette will do."

About 9:00 P.M. that night, the trade was made and I lay alone in bed and smoked the joint. I knew there was a possibility that members of the hospital staff might be able to smell the aroma of burning cannabis coming from my room, but at that point in time I was hurting too much to care. What the hell did I have to lose, anyway?

Fifteen minutes after smoking that joint I picked up the phone and dialed the nurse station, begging for solid food. It was the first time I had experienced an appetite in a month.

Shortly thereafter, two nurses arrived carrying a plate of very lean roast beef, covered with gravy and steaming hot. The nurses only took two steps into the room before I knew I couldn't eat what they brought; the smell instantly racked my stomach with intense nausea.

When I protested, the nurses asked me what I wanted and I ordered raw vegetables and fruit. This wasn't an easy order to fill in the middle of a harsh Iowa winter. The nurses argued that they felt I needed to have protein and they feared that I wouldn't be strong enough to chew the raw fruit and vegetables.

Once I convinced the nurses that I absolutely could not eat unless they brought me something I found palatable and digestible, I prevailed in the debate. A few minutes later a bowl of raw carrots, celery and cauliflower appeared. I devoured it slowly and deliberately, as I had to chew the food into tiny pieces before swallowing it. I ate like my life depended on it, which it did. Then I ordered vanilla ice cream and chocolate milkshakes. Throughout the night, I slept soundly for the first time in six weeks, waking up only one time to order more ice cream. I also ate a regular breakfast the next morning with eggs, bacon and hash browns, served hospital style.

I could barely believe it. Was it really possible that a tattoo, a joint and a cancer patient had rescued me, just moments away from my doctor-ordained hour of death?

My kind beneficiary from down the hall, who was evidently extremely addicted to tobacco, died three days later. Though I never met him, I offer him my heartfelt gratitude for serving as a messenger at a time I direly needed one. His final act of compassion saved my life. For this I give thanks to the anonymous friend I never knew.

I immediately began repeating my request to leave the hospital, but my doctors were still very worried about my ability to survive. I must have driven them insane with my constant pleas. They spent hours searching my medical charts and records for any indicator or correlation that could explain the abrupt halt in the progression of my symptoms, but they were eventually forced to admit they were stumped. The hospital physicians finally promised me that if I could live an entire week, until the weekend, while maintaining my eating and sleeping throughout this period of time, then they would consider letting me go home.

I patiently and persistently jumped through their hoops, but as Saturday approached my doctors still didn't think I could live through the long trip home. When Saturday arrived I rolled my hospital appliances, monitors and other machinery attached to me up and down the shiny halls to visit each doctor's office individually. Much to the consternation of my physicians, I voluntarily signed paperwork stating that I was checking myself out of that damned hospital, against their medical advice, thus releasing the doctors from any legal responsibility for the consequences of my actions.

By 7:00 P.M. that evening, I was fully checked out of the hospital and lying in the back of a beat-up station wagon my wife had borrowed from a friend. Margaret drove us home through a blinding snowstorm, the wipers tapping out a fragile heartbeat on the half-frozen windshield, while I tried to stay focused and relaxed with my children lovingly nursing me in the cargo area.

I hadn't been outside of the hospital in over three months. My body seemed to register every bump and crack in the road as we flew down the highway, jolting me with sharp twinges of pain. Although the long drive was hard on my body, it felt so good just to be outside, to be traveling somewhere, away from white coats, loud intercoms and filthy bedpans. That trip home was 250 miles of throbbing agony and sheer ecstasy.

As we drove home, I shared the details of my survival with my family. I continued to suspect that marijuana had saved my life. Yet it seemed too ridiculous to be true. I racked my brain for some other explanation, but try as I might, there was simply no tangible reason why I'd suddenly regained my appetite. I held on to my pain pills, however, just in case I was mistaken.

Providence visited me again on the morning after I arrived home from the hospital. I was worn out from the drive and I'd just begun adjusting to the reality of being home when a sharp knock came at the front door. It was Greg, a younger friend of mine, and a couple of his party buddies. They wanted an old car that I had sitting in my backyard and they'd brought a paper grocery bag, filled to the top with low-quality ditch weed, to trade for it.

It was strange serendipity. These guys had no idea that I needed marijuana for medicine. However, the timing of their request was impeccable.

After I invited them inside, I smoked a large joint. Even though the quality of the weed was rough, it helped me to feel better. Greg showed me how to increase the potency of the marijuana by a primitive process of alcohol extraction. All they had was five pounds of weed, two-fifths of Everclear alcohol, one big bowl, one nylon stocking and one light bulb. The weeklong process was straightforward: soak, strain, remove, evaporate and scrape. Simple ingredients and a simple method. More importantly, it made a big difference.

A week later I smoked a joint of the strengthened herb and found my suspicions about its positive effects on my weak body were immediately confirmed. Marijuana was definitely improving my health and well-being in obvious ways: it eased my pain and nausea, relieved my spasms and stimulated my appetite.

That evening, I threw away all my pain medication. It wasn't an impulsive leap of faith anymore; I was certain that marijuana was medicine. The pills, tablets and capsules looked like pharmaceutical confetti as they swirled down the commode and out of my life.

As my health began to improve, I was eager to embrace life again. This included reestablishing my relationship with my wife. I hadn't seen my wife for ninety days while I was recuperating in the hospital. By the time I returned home, my barbarian soul ached for the virtuous love of my beautiful wife, my Queen Margaret.

I learned there was an irritating drawback to this rejuvenated sense of passion. My body simply could not accomplish what my heart and mind wished for. I was a self-certified Don Juan turned Don Quixote. It was really difficult for me to accept any sexual limitations. Once I got through that stubborn stage, however, I discovered that with creative imagination I could redefine my personal experience of sex and adapt accordingly.

Although I was in a depleted state and barely able to move, I was still alive with desire. I was sure of it, because I felt a raging need for human contact. After some serious forethought, my wife and I completed our sacred mission. Margaret was glorious and sleep was finally attained.

Sex is a core issue for most chronically ill people, but it's not often spoken of at cocktail parties. It makes many patients very uncomfortable to discuss the matter, particularly with healthy, virile people who take for granted the physical and emotional rewards of truly passionate sex. Who wants to think about being so ill you must give up making love?

Over the years I've talked with several young, able-bodied people who naively assume that disease and disability cause patients to lose the natural longing for sex. This may be true in some cases, but many patients discover that they actually experience an increase in sexual desire. In a way, it makes sense. After all, good sex with a loving partner affirms the body, heals the heart and exalts the spirit. Nothing feels better than howling in the face of death and many patients, especially those gravely ill, desperately need to feel intensely alive in the here and now.

I continued to smoke cannabis illegally over the next two years. I knew this was a major risk, but the threat of a lonely prison cell paled in comparison with the cold darkness of the grave. I was determined to do almost anything to stay alive and mitigate the severity of my symptoms, even if it meant being called a criminal by some misguided people.

It was rough to deal with being labeled a lawbreaker, but I got through it because I always knew that in an ethical sense, I was no criminal. I was simply a human being in a bizarre circumstance, caught between the letter and spirit of the law.

Using illegal marijuana to ease my pain had distinct, critical disadvantages. For one thing, I could never rely on a steady supply of herb. A million different things might happen. The dealer could run out of marijuana, money or luck. I might travel all the way across town to discover that the dealer had disappeared or been arrested. It wasn't like I could phone in my prescription ahead of time and most dealers don't keep regular business hours or make house calls. Obtaining the medicine I needed so badly was a hit and miss activity.

Assuming my dealer was home and had marijuana, the only acceptable form of payment was cash. No checks and no plastic. In response to strict government drug policies and stiff legal penalties, prices were high, running anywhere from $25-45 per quarter ounce of weed. Most sick and disabled people have a hard enough time making ends meet without paying the exorbitant prices of black market medicine, but the only other choice was getting sicker and going without relief.

Another major problem once I had my cannabis in hand, was that there was no way to ensure it would be of acceptable quality. For example, some marijuana is transported in cases of incense that mask the smell of the illegal herb. This makes for terrible smoking after the incense dust particles mix with the medicine. Some marijuana isn't stored properly, gets damp and becomes covered in mold. This fungus isn't a problem for patients with a healthy immune system, but inhaling certain types of spores could cause a potentially fatal lung infection in AIDS patients or others, like myself, with suppressed immune systems.

Furthermore, in order to obtain my medicine safely, I had to distinguish between who was trustworthy and who was not. I found it was no simple task to navigate the vast and covert networks of the criminal underworld. Although there are dealers who care about their product and the people to whom they sell it, many are unscrupulous and will do anything to increase their profit margins. Some dealers even mix their pot with oregano, catnip or other spices, just so they can rip people off. Dishonesty thrives in an unregulated underground market and, ultimately, dealers are accountable to no one but themselves.

Legal ramifications were also a major concern. The person selling my medicine could be an undercover police officer or could be a criminal turned informant working for the police. Narcotics officers often use a single bust to then ensnare an entire chain of people and some dealers, when faced with the threat of prosecution, are quick to cooperate with the demands of police, even if it means setting up their friends and customers—whether those friends and customers are occasional recreational users or very sick individuals using the herb for medicinal purposes.

I had to inspect my herb carefully when I got it from people I didn't know, sifting it through my fingers to check the grade and smell. If it's tainted with other drugs or products, it could make you ill. Unfortunately, you can't just show up at the emergency room if you get sick from somebody selling you bad marijuana. If you try to seek medical attention, you might find yourself wheeled out of the hospital in a pair of handcuffs. And although physician informants were extremely rare at that time, the media made a mountain out of a molehill, repeatedly reporting any instance of marijuana-using patients ensnared by police with doctors' help to espouse propaganda regarding the dangers of cannabis use.

Finally, if upon sampling my medicine I was dissatisfied with the purchase, there was no refund or exchange. There were also no receipts. Most dealers would have laughed at any buyer asking for his or her money back. There was nobody to file a civil action against. There was also no bureau or regulatory committee to complain to, except the police. Any patient who filed a report was liable to be either detained by the cops or shot by the dealers, only to become another statistical victim of a senseless drug policy.

While smoking an equivalent of ten marijuana cigarettes

per day, I was as comfortable as possible and didn't require the strong prescribed medications or the surgeries. My family and friends witnessed a radical transformation in my health.

Occasionally, friends asked me if I ever got high from smoking black market pot. It was difficult to make them understand. First of all, I had to get them to clarify what they meant by "high." I certainly didn't feel inebriated or dull-headed. I didn't walk around in a stoned, lethargic stupor. I didn't wail and guffaw at terrible jokes or philosophize about the linoleum floor in my kitchen. My response to marijuana simply did not fit the prevalent stereotype of "getting high."

People who have never struggled with a life threatening or disabling illness often do not comprehend how debilitating the resulting depression can be. Long days spent struggling with sickness can wear patients down, suppress their appetites and slowly destroy their wills to live. This psychological damage can result in physiological effects that may be the difference between living and dying.

The elevated mood associated with cannabis definitely affected my health in a positive manner. I was more engaged with life. I took walks and rode my bike, things I never considered doing before in my depressed state, even if I had been physically capable. I ate regular meals and I slept better at night. All of these individual factors contributed to a better overall sense of well-being.

If you feel better, you are better. For many people, this may seem obvious, but for me it was a discovery that changed the way I thought about my illness. I accepted the fact that I might not ever be cured of my condition, but at least I had found a way to feel less physical and emotional pain in the meantime.

Because it was so beneficial to my quality of life, I began to consider what might happen if I fully divulged the fact of my cannabis use to all of my physicians. Some of them might disapprove and advise me against it. Still, it was a risk I felt I had to take. After all, this was my life at stake. If I couldn't talk about this to the people who were providing me with medical care, who could I talk to?

Much to my surprise, I rarely found a doctor who wasn't willing to listen when I shared my story and most of them empathized with my dilemma. They never called me a drug addict and they never turned me in to the police. Some of the physicians agreed that cannabis was having medical benefits for me, but conveyed that they felt powerless to do anything about it. They all said the same thing: they weren't in positions where they could take a public stand on the issue of legalizing medical marijuana.

Some of these doctors tried to offer me traditional therapies to supplement my use of cannabis smoking. Although I appreciated the significant gains brought about by medical innovation, I told my physicians that in the past I'd suffered too many side effects which dehumanized me and that I wanted to avoid pharmaceutical and surgical treatments if I could. The doctors meant well, but they had been trained to react to illness by prescribing pills or slicing into my body. For me, these traditional remedies weren't worth the substantial risks involved. Every time I felt waves of pain coming on, it reminded me of the multiple ways in which misguided practitioners had violated my body.

Despite my protestations, my doctors and their staffs continued to seek treatment options for me considered acceptable within the medical establishment. One nurse at the university hospital went so far as to write to over three hundred doctors' offices in five states to see if any of them could treat Nail Patella Syndrome. Finally, she received one answer to her inquiry. The nurse was so excited about this response that she tracked me down at the hospital pain clinic to tell me that she found a doctor who was willing to treat me.

Although I reiterated that I didn't want pills or unnecessary treatments, I agreed to look into this new option before dismissing it outright. However, I was concerned that the doctor might be located several states away. I couldn't believe there would be a doctor close to where I presently lived and my family and I feared we'd have to move. When the nurse located the doctor's address, I was elated to discover that his office was only twenty miles from my home.

I went to see this new doctor the following week. When I arrived, I learned his office was in the very hospital in which I was born thirty-eight years earlier. Although the faces of staff had changed, these were the same buildings I started life in. I felt like I had come full circle.

From the moment we first met, my new doctor and nurse treated me as if we were all part of the same big family. They were aware that I was using marijuana and they were open to the idea that marijuana worked as medicine to alleviate pain for me. In fact, they were prepared to do whatever it took to find a way for me to legally use marijuana. My new nurse took on all of the essential paperwork duties working in tandem with my new doctor.

Initially, my doctor applied to the state government's Board of Pharmacy to seek approval to prescribe marijuana to his patient. The board immediately responded, "We would love to approve this!" Four days later, he received a second message. This time the board said it made a mistake and could not approve my use of medical marijuana; we had to apply to the federal government.

In the meantime, my wife found a magazine article about Elvy Musikka, a glaucoma patient who was the third legal marijuana recipient in the United States. I got in touch with Elvy and told her my story and about my doctor's efforts on my behalf to apply to become a legal medical marijuana recipient. Elvy spoke passionately about the program and how it saved her life, but she warned me becoming approved would be a long, arduous process. She advised me to get in touch with Robert Randall, the first legal medical marijuana patient, because he could tell me exactly what I needed to do. After dialing the number Elvy gave me, I heard the voice of Robert Randall come on the line. He listened to my story and enthusiastically agreed to help me apply to become part of the program he helped to get started. He gave me the reference numbers for the federal medical forms my doctor would need to submit in order to obtain an Investigational New Drug Protocol, which would then allow me to smoke marijuana legally.

I passed along the reference numbers for the necessary forms to my doctor who ordered them from the government. A few weeks later they arrived. My doctor and I reviewed them together to be sure we could provide all the documentation and proof that was required. Much to my relief, my doctor and his nurse both thought it could be done, so I signed a form that allowed my doctor to begin the application process.

My nurse and doctor started from scratch, researching relevant contact information and filing extensive paperwork with the Drug Enforcement Agency (DEA), the National Institute on Drug Abuse (NIDA) and the Food and Drug Administration (FDA) over and over again for two years. The filings included three forms, one page each, and forty pages of protocol description, detailing the specifics of my medical history and what marijuana was expected to do for me.

My doctor and nurse were still uncertain of the specific medical benefits of cannabis, but they knew that I was having less pain, spasms and nausea, and my intake of pharmaceutical drugs decreased with no other changes in my treatment besides the use of marijuana. They were not sure what the outcome of the application process would eventually be. The only things they were sure about were that I was being helped by marijuana and my health status fulfilled the medical prerequisites for the federal protocol.

My doctor encountered many problems with the application process. For one thing, the federal forms had to be filled out absolutely perfectly. A simple mistake like a period left off the end of a sentence or a typo could make authorities throw my paperwork in the trashcan, where it would promptly be forgotten. My doctor only found this out weeks later when he called government officials to verify my application status.

My doctor requested that I stop smoking marijuana. He wished to observe any physiological changes that coincided with the removal of cannabis from my system. He also believed that I had a better chance of being accepted into the federal marijuana program if we had hard clinical data demonstrating both the physical deterioration that occurred when I stopped smoking marijuana and the restorative effects of the drug when I resumed use of it.

The way my doctor explained it, I was in a catch-22. I wouldn't get the marijuana if the federal bureaucrats thought I was too healthy, but if I was too sick I might die before they approved me for the program. In my opinion, some of those bureaucrats would have preferred to see me "go gentle into the good night," just to avoid making any waves. They obviously didn't know me very well.

In the end, I was forced to quit smoking marijuana for several months. I had to be a guinea pig for the federal government, just to ensure there was absolutely no way for officials to deny the extent of my suffering and deterioration. I felt like the government officials were making me jump through hoops covered with razors, doused in gasoline and set aflame. It was not an easy proposition to accept, especially when I was sure I would become so sick again.

However, I was prepared to do whatever it took to get legal access to effective medicine, so I stopped smoking. The symptoms were immediately evident and progressive. Within weeks I was in uncontrollable pain and within months I was progressively terminal again.

I resumed taking a variety of pharmaceutical medications to control and alleviate my symptoms. I took so many pills I could have made a meal of them. In fact, one night, I nearly choked on them. There were enough pills to fill my queasy stomach, but I sure couldn't live this way.

In fact, I was up to seventeen different pills, three times a day and I was pretty incapacitated because of the side effects when my application was finally approved and my doctor received my first shipment of medical marijuana from the federal government.

Nevertheless, I felt elated when that supply of legal cannabis was actually in my hands. The doctor allowed me to open the first can. I pulled off the lid of the silver can with my aching fingers, and gazed down at three hundred government joints. He handed me one dose (a single joint). I left his office, smoked the joint and returned a short while later. He asked me if the medicine worked, if I felt better, and I replied that it had and I did. He smiled and handed me nine more doses of medical marijuana, wrapped in paper tubes, to be smoked that day. He told me he would see me the next morning.

This routine continued daily for weeks, with the period between in-person check-ups gradually lengthening. Eventually I was able to make one personal visit to my doctor every four months in order to obtain my medication.

I struggled long and hard to reach this milestone. Many people said it couldn't be done. However, after all those years of fighting, I finally won.

||| 4
Bureaucrats for Prison, Politicians for Prozac

*No one can make you feel inferior
without your consent.*

– Eleanor Roosevelt

Finally, our small caravan arrives in Little Rock, Arkansas. We go to our hotel and, since it's late, we all head straight to our rooms for a good night's sleep.

In the morning, we meet Arkansas State Senator John Riggs for breakfast at a local café. I tell the senator about how medical marijuana has helped me. I tell him that I don't want to see another sick or dying person live in needless pain or in fear of being arrested and the only way to get it legalized is with congressional support. He listens, empathizes and promises that he will do what he can to support a bill toward the legalization of medical marijuana.

I leave the café feeling upbeat; the discussion went well and it appears we have another state legislator on our side. I smile at Margaret who squeezes my hand reassuringly. She knows I soon face another major hurdle this morning.

We arrive at the state capitol building a few minutes later. The documentary team waits for us on the lawn while Margaret, Christopher and I head in. We are soon ushered into the tastefully decorated office of the Arkansas State Capitol Police Chief, Richard H. Peterson. I stand in front of his desk, in my hands a sealed, silver can containing three hundred marijuana joints given to me by the federal government. I'm wearing my finest clothes and a broad smile.

Margaret sits quietly in a leather chair behind me, my steady port in a stormy sea. She has been through this with me many times before and knows the ropes, so she is familiar with the process and calmly bides her time.

Christopher is not so sure as he shuffles his weight from foot to foot. He stands beside me, wearing a dashing black suit, complete with a fedora hat, which he does not remove. He comes from the new school, where it's not considered disrespectful to leave your hat on indoors. Some friends have said he looks like one of the Blues Brothers without the sunglasses. Standing six feet, three inches tall, many people think he is my bodyguard and I like it that way. Not to be paranoid, but I never know when somebody might try to take me on.

Chief Peterson is a handsome, broad-shouldered man who appears to be in his mid-fifties. Dressed in a tailored brown suit, he sits behind a large mahogany desk. He does not look amused.

"Mr. McMahon, I appreciate you notifying us in advance of your intent to visit."

"No problem. I want to do everything possible to avoid any trouble for you and your men."

The chief wrinkles his brow as he wrings his leathery hands. "Since the time we last spoke, our officers have literally made hundreds of phone calls. We've contacted the DEA, the FDA and the National Institute of Drug Abuse. Some officials at these agencies had no idea the federal government was growing marijuana. Others stated they were aware of the Compassionate IND Program, but they thought it no longer existed. Still others knew there were patients still receiving the marijuana, but they wouldn't give out any names. The left hand doesn't know what the right hand is doing."

I shake my head and sigh. "I've run into this problem before. They won't provide information about us because it will violate our medical privacy and make them vulnerable to a lawsuit."

"Do you have some kind of identification that can prove your legal status?"

"Sure, I've got my card from the Oakland Cannabis Buyers' Cooperative in California. I've got newspaper clippings of articles about me from all over the country. I've got copies of my medical protocol." I stoop down, reach into my briefcase and hand him a stack of papers.

The chief takes a minute to look over the paperwork and then hands the papers back to me. "Unfortunately, this doesn't give me what I need, Mr. McMahon. The card from California is not legally binding here in Arkansas. I've got to have papers from the federal government, something that serves as proof of your right to smoke marijuana in our state."

"There's no ID system for members of the Compassionate IND Program."

Chief Peterson sighs deeply and shakes his head.

I stand before him, not really knowing what to say, thinking about this insane impasse. How frustrating it is for me. How crazy it must seem to the chief. We are two men caught in an absurd whirlwind of law and politics.

Chief Peterson can arrest me right here and now, since I've brought a substantial amount of marijuana into the state capitol building and he has no legal proof that I have the right to do so. Instead of dancing to the jailhouse rock at Graceland, where we will be going tomorrow, I could be spending several nights holed up in a cell, tossing back and forth on a chilly concrete slab, without any medicine to numb my pain or help me sleep. Rather than speaking at the University of Mississippi, as I'm scheduled to do this week, I could be struggling to keep from throwing up my lunch, without my marijuana, as if jailhouse grub wasn't bad enough. My green path might dead end at a brick wall with steel bars.

On the other hand, if the chief decides to incarcerate me, he'll be taking the risk that I might just actually be who I say I am. My wife, my co-author and a documentary crew will be working overtime, busy getting the word out to hungry reporters. By the time officials are able to verify my legal status, Chief Peterson could be doing his best to cope with some very negative national media coverage.

In a very real sense, we are at each other's mercy...

The room is hot and stuffy and my back is starting to hurt from standing for so long. I kneel on the floor on one knee, still looking the chief in the eye. He seems like a good man who is just trying to do his job without violating the law he is sworn to uphold.

After thinking about the situation for a moment, I speak. "It's a shame that you have to go through all this. You're probably used to dealing with these situations on a state level. In the federal realm, things can get kind of hectic."

"Well, I'm sure finding that out."

"I wish it were different," I tell him. "That's why I had breakfast with Senator Riggs this morning. If sick and dying people in your state could use marijuana to control or alleviate their pain and symptoms without the threat of arrest, these problems could be avoided."

The police chief nods sympathetically. "I hope you understand that to me, this issue isn't about marijuana. It's about medicine. I don't like to have to play politics with health. I care about people dealing with painful illnesses and I have no desire to arrest a sick person. But my hands are still tied by our state laws."

"I understand. It's a difficult position you're in."

Chief Peterson looks directly into my eyes, trying to get a feel for who I am. "We called some other state capitols that you visited in the past—Iowa, Texas, Minnesota. Officials there all said you are good to your word."

I look into his eyes to size him up. "I'm flattered they hold me in such high regard, Chief. I'm not here to make trouble, but I do want to see your state law changed."

Chief Peterson pauses. "We've got another problem. A few days ago, I received a copy of an E-mail that's been circulating throughout our legislative offices claiming that you intend to light a joint on the front steps of the capitol during your press conference."

Shaking my head, I respond, "I don't know anything about that. I didn't write that E-mail and I don't know who did. I never told anybody I would smoke on the capitol steps. I assure you, I only smoke when I need to."

"I know the reporters want their money shot for the front pages," Peterson sighs, "but if you light up on the capitol steps, then I'm going to get dozens of phone calls from angry citizens insisting that I enforce the state code and arrest you. I wouldn't want to do that for anything in the world, Mr. McMahon, but I don't currently have any legal grounds to let me off the hook on this one. I'm going to ask that if you need to smoke marijuana while you are here, do it discreetly. We won't be following you around the capitol grounds. There are plenty of places where you can take your medicine if you need it."

"That sounds fine. I want you to know, I have no intention of insulting or disgracing you in your own town. I'll still open the can and take a joint out for the cameras, but I won't turn it into a media sideshow act."

"Well, I want this event to be good for everybody, so I appreciate your working with me on this one. By the way, one of our men will attend your press conference on the steps, but that is our blanket policy for all press conferences, as a security service."

Smiling, I rise and offer my hand to the chief. He takes it.

Christopher picks up and carries my heavy, brown leather briefcase as he and Margaret follow me out of the chief's office into the foyer of the state capitol, past the armed guards and metal detectors and out the doors to the capitol lawn. The fresh air smells good. I am free again, but after all the physical and mental stress, I really need a joint.

My wife and friend give me just the kind of unspoken but affirming support I need. I prefer to handle these bureaucratic quagmires for myself whenever I possibly can, but the presence of people who care about me means a great deal whenever I am in a difficult situation.

The looming dome of the capitol building dwarfs the three of us as we shuffle along. A warm wind gusts up the long front steps that lead down to the statues and green grass of the capitol lawn. I grab my marijuana can tightly to ensure it doesn't get blown away. There's something immensely satisfying about being able to walk this path with three hundred legal joints in my hand.

We meet up with the documentary team and Christopher tells them how it went with Chief Peterson. I smile at Margaret, knowing that with a government joint, a little luck and two balls of steel, I just might make it through the rest of the day without being cuffed and booked for breaking a law that doesn't apply to me and the few other American citizens who legally smoke Uncle Sam's marijuana.

We slowly walk a half-block away from the capitol, to the Capitol Hill building that houses both offices and apartments for legislators, where I am scheduled to speak at a congressional luncheon sponsored by Justice of the Peace Wilandra Dean. The event was organized in preparation for a medical marijuana bill that will soon be authored in Arkansas.

To many politicians I'm a living contradiction, the dysfunctional functional. When I visit their offices, I'm often a complete enigma to them. By the time I leave, I'm either their best friend or their worst nightmare.

Christopher, Margaret and I step through the front doors into a posh, carpeted lobby where roughly two-dozen people mill about several tables that are adorned with snacks and literature on medical marijuana. I'm hungry, but I'm too keyed-up to eat right now, so I pass by the food to greet my fellow citizens, supporters and detractors. As my right hand is severely disabled, I hope they don't mind me shaking with my left hand.

Even with the presence of detractors, there are no enemies here, only supporters and potential allies. It's a diverse group of legislators, reporters, activists, doctors and, most importantly, patients. Congressional members in attendance include Representatives Jan Judy of Fayetteville, Joyce Dees of Warren and Shirley Borhauer of Benton County.

Several reporters from publications and media outlets including the *Arkansas Democrat-Gazette*, the Associated Press, the Donrey Media Group, the *Little Rock Free Press* and the local National Public Radio affiliate have gathered to cover the luncheon.

Two patients who illegally use medical marijuana have demonstrated great bravery by attending this event: John Markes, a Vietnam veteran and medical marijuana user who suffers from a rare form of wasting syndrome, and Van Spence, a quadriplegic man who uses marijuana to treat his pain and spasms. They both make appearances in spite of the fact that public disclosures of their marijuana use could be the catalysts for their investigations and arrests. Courageous patients such as these two men are an inspiration to me and the ultimate reason I continue to try and teach people about the importance and necessity of legalizing medical marijuana.

Dr. Carl Covey, a Little Rock pain specialist who is an active member of the American Medical Association, has come at the request of a representative who was not able to attend and who had pledged to send twenty doctors to refute every fact I assert. Only one doctor actually showed up.

I get excited when doctors come to these events, because even if some of them believe that smoking marijuana is bad medicine, their presence implies a desire to engage in the dialogue. As scientists, they are willing to consider the possibility that marijuana actually helps sick people.

My legs are weak from all the walking, so I sit down in a comfortable, cushioned chair in the corner. A large, burly man with long, flowing silver hair and a scraggly beard approaches me with his hand extended. Looking like a cross between Tolstoy and Santa Claus, he certainly stands out from the rest of the crowd.

He shakes my left hand and says, "Hello. Are you George?"

"That's me," I respond simply. I make no inquiry of him. In fact, I hardly ever ask people what group they represent or are associated with, because I really don't care. I just want to talk with people one-on-one. I figure this guy must be an activist.

"I'm Representative Jim Lendall. I'm a congressman here at the state capitol."

Wow, I think. *I wasn't expecting that!* Another wild guess effectively debunked.

"Well, I'm glad you could make it, Jim. You're supporting the upcoming medical marijuana bill, aren't you?"

"I sure am. In addition to being a congressman, I'm a full-time nurse and I've seen with my own eyes the wonders cannabis works for some patients. I think the way our state treats sick and dying people is absolutely criminal and I want to thank you for coming here to speak."

I am delighted by Jim's candor. "I hope my visit can help affect some change."

He nods encouragingly.

The moderator calls the room to order. Our eclectic group is gathered into a large seated circle for a question and answer session, while organizers hand out chicken salad sandwiches to the attendees. It's hard to eat and talk at the same time and I no longer have an appetite, so I pass on the sandwich and focus on the task at hand.

After a brief introduction, I offer a few opening remarks and then the debate begins. Dr. Covey is the first guest to engage in debate and he speaks with intense deliberation, weighing his words carefully. He is skeptical about the medical efficacy of marijuana and he knows he's got a tough audience. One thing is for sure, he's got guts.

"Mr. McMahon, how would you address the potential for diversion of medical marijuana to the black market if it were to be decriminalized?"

"To be perfectly honest, doctor, I don't address it at all," I respond. "Diversion is an issue for the police. I try to focus on medicine. As a patient, health is the relevant matter to me."

"Diversion is a very real problem for the medical community, Mr. McMahon. Aside from the legal aspect, it impacts health if somebody is taking an unregulated drug that they shouldn't be taking."

"I think you are right about that, Doctor Covey. It certainly impacts health. Even now, pharmaceutical substances like Xanax, Ritalin and Valium get diverted every day. We have law enforcement officials who are well trained to specifically focus on the problem. But we don't criminalize the sick people who legitimately use Xanax, just because some others forge fake prescriptions or sell the drug on the black market. I'm here to talk about patients, not criminals."

"Okay, let's discuss the patients. How do you respond, George, to the numerous studies that indicate there are negative health consequences to smoking marijuana?"

I clear my throat. "With all due respect, doctor, those studies are critically flawed. For one thing, they are not replicable, which as you know is one of the crucial criteria for acceptable scientific research. And most of the studies, since they are sponsored by government agencies, are not impartial. They're designed from the outset to find harm. They aren't looking for medical benefits in the first place, so of course they don't find any."

Dr. Covey leans forward slightly. "Well I think one of the problems is that all the evidence is anecdotal. The medical community just doesn't have enough empirical data to warrant the release of a potentially dangerous drug. If you want the medical community to support your cause, you've got to demonstrate proof."

"I've already got that proof. I can show you dozens of solid, replicable studies that were overlooked and suppressed by government officials and members of the mainstream media. In fact, I recently participated in a longitudinal study that focused on chronic cannabis use in the Compassionate Investigational New Drug Program, which assessed benefits and adverse effects of legal, clinical cannabis. This is the only research study on the legal patients, like myself, that has been published in over twenty-four years of the federal program's existence."

Dr. Covey shakes his head and says, "I haven't seen this study so I wouldn't be able to comment on it."

I reach over and sift through a stack of manila file folders I have brought that are laid out on the table in front of me. When I find the folder I'm looking for, I point to it and say, "Well, I have a study on the subject right here. You're more than welcome to take a copy with you if you like. This study found that long-term and extensive use of cannabis may cause some cognitive impairment, but the numerous physiological benefits outweigh the minor cognitive implications."

Christopher, who is sitting right next to Dr. Covey, turns to him and adds, "The cognitive impairment associated with long-term marijuana use is insignificant when compared with the cognitive effects of powerful drugs like morphine, Demerol, codeine, and Valium."

John Markes leans forward, resting his elbows on the arms of his wheelchair. He turns to Dr. Covey and says, "Besides, I don't think that people who are dying of cancer or AIDS are really that concerned with the minor cognitive impact of smoking an herb that is not only adding months to their lives, but easing their symptoms and pain."

Several chuckles come from the crowd. It's hard to argue with a person in a wheelchair, but I can empathize with Dr. Covey, nevertheless. After all, there was a time in my life when I basically believed the same myths. I think he is the only person in the room who does not support marijuana as medicine. I imagine he is feeling very conscious of his minority status right now, but I feel everyone has room to grow.

Dr. Covey glances from person to person and says, "What about the delivery system? I mean, there probably isn't a doctor out there who would argue that marijuana has absolutely *no* medicinal properties whatsoever, but I know there are many physicians who have legitimate concerns about patients smoking *any* type of medicine. There are fears that the long-term smoking of cannabis may have detrimental effects to the lung tissue."

"But you see, doctor, smoking is actually the most effective method of taking my medicine. Smoked cannabis is absorbed through my lungs. The effects are relatively instant and this allows me to regulate my dosage in a very precise manner. I don't have that kind of control when I eat marijuana."

"What about the pharmaceutical alternatives like Marinol?"

"I think there should be alternative delivery systems, particularly for those patients with respiratory problems. However, I don't think Marinol will work for me. One of the reasons I smoke marijuana is to treat my nausea. Swallowing a concentrated dose of synthetic THC could make me even more nauseous. I will make one concession, though. If the pharmaceutical companies create a delivery system that is just as effective as smoking, without the potential drawbacks, I will be happy to try it."

Dr. Covey pauses for a moment, then says earnestly, "I'll come right out and state that I am not a supporter of medical marijuana. I do think it is extremely important, however, to acknowledge that compassionate people stand on both sides of this issue and people on both sides care about the patients. If we don't recognize that, then we have an obstacle from the start. I know there are good doctors working with the American Medical Association and they care deeply about extending life and relieving the suffering of these patients. We may have to agree to disagree on specific points, but we can still find common ground to work with."

"I could not agree with you more, doctor. There are good people on both sides, but a great deal of harm can be done in the name of helping. If we really care about patients, we should be listening to them. What do people with cancer, AIDS, glaucoma, MS, spinal cord injury and Nail Patella Syndrome think about medical marijuana? Why do we dismiss their medical experiences as merely anecdotal? We should be including that feedback in our deliberation. True compassion demands that we listen. After all, we hear politicians, pundits and law enforcement officials talking about this health issue all the time. I know a lot of patients and doctors who have trouble being heard above the discord."

As Dr. Covey considers my point, I feel like there is a hint of revelation in his eyes. He may be more of an ally than he realizes. After all, he is posing the types of challenging questions that will inevitably be asked at the federal level, so he is giving medical marijuana advocates an opportunity to prepare themselves in a safe, relatively informal setting. I don't expect him to start handing out joints to his patients anytime in the near future, but I can see he is beginning to sort out the tangled mess of legal, medical and political issues.

After a few more questions and comments, our debate comes to an end. People stand up and mill about, discussing the issues and finishing their lunches. I always try to give my audience just enough to leave them wanting to know more. I hope people will pursue more research on their own time, after I'm long gone. If I've inspired them to do that, I've accomplished my goal.

The questions haven't been antagonistic this time, but there have been a few occasions when I've spoken that individuals in the audience were verbally abusive and tried to heckle me.

During a press conference a few years earlier, one particular woman repeatedly tried to make me look foolish in front of an audience that included the Public Safety Commissioner, the

Health Commissioner, the Governor of Minnesota and a representative from every state law enforcement agency. The heckler was a mature woman, wearing a light blue business suit and glasses. She reminded me of my sweet grandmother, until she opened her mouth.

In front of the large crowd, she asked me, "Do you think we should give pot to children?"

I leaned back in my chair for just a moment and then said, "If the child has a serious illness or disability and marijuana will help that child have a better quality of life, then you bet I support giving him or her marijuana, just like any other medication that could help a child."

Unappeased, the woman then asked, "Would you actually let your grandkids sit on your lap while you smoke a joint?"

I responded, "You know, it's not really any of your business where my grandkids sit." The entire audience snickered at her failed attempt to lower me to her level.

The woman sat silent for a few seconds before stooping even lower. I've found this kind of attack is common for people who don't have any facts to stand behind. They naturally resort to personal attacks. She said, "Why does your voice sound so funny? Is it because you smoke so much dope?"

I took a deep breath and placed my arms on the table in front of me. "No. I have many friends and family members who have known me for decades and they can attest that since I was young man my voice has always sounded rough and gravely. Nice try, though."

My mind snaps back to the present. Fortunately, the questions at today's conference were thoughtful. Admittedly, I was still being forced to distinguish between medical and recreational use of marijuana, but that's a tough issue for many people to really grasp, unless they are patients.

I walk outside and cross the street, moving toward the capitol. My body aches and I wish I had time to smoke a joint, but I'm scheduled to speak at a press conference in five minutes. *It's okay,* I tell myself. *I can take the pain for a little while longer.*

As I make my way toward the front steps of the capitol, a long chain of representatives, journalists, activists and patients follow me. For one fleeting moment I feel like the Pied Piper of Hamelin, but I know that I have no disciples. If I ever found out that people were calling themselves my followers, I'd tell them to bug off and think for themselves. That's what makes this country great and what helps to get issues discussed—independent thought.

As I step up to the podium on the steps of the capitol building, in front of several photographers, video cameras and wheelchairs, I notice a fully uniformed police officer standing quietly nearby. Just as Chief Peterson promised, the state capitol police have provided me with security during the press conference. Some of the more radical activists in the crowd might assume the officer is here to ensure that nobody smokes marijuana at the capitol building, but I know he's here to protect my freedom of speech.

I'm amazed to see Chief Peterson step out of his office and walk over to the uniformed officer. The chief stands quietly next to the officer. Now that I think about it, maybe I'm not so amazed that he wants to hear what I'm going to say. If I had a dollar for every officer who's kept an open mind when it comes to medical cannabis, I would be a wealthy man. Perhaps they are caught between the letter and the spirit of the law as much as anyone else.

I pull the microphone toward my lips and glance behind me at the capitol dome soaring overhead. Turning back to the crowd, I move closer to the podium, prepared to lean on it if I start having intense pain. If I have to, I'll sit right down on the steps of the capitol and finish my speech from a squatting position. I just hope the journalists are willing to meet me at my own level.

A gust of wind tosses my hair about. I clear my throat and begin to speak. "Much of the crowd assembled here today represents the beliefs and wishes of half a million people. Each person here represents about ten thousand Americans, maybe more. Americans who want medical marijuana legalized.

"Despite some rumors, I would like you to know I did not come here to smoke marijuana on the steps of your capitol. I came here to respectfully ask members of your legislature to honor your wishes.

"Several legislators who are on our side of this issue have commented that what they need is your support, so we want you to let them know you are behind them. We already know that sixty percent of the people in Arkansas believe marijuana could be useful medicine and patients should have access to it. Sixty percent of you will come out and say it, but how many more of you are afraid to do that? We think one hundred percent of you would support it if you felt like you could and that is why we are here today.

"You need to tell your representative and senator how you feel. You need to go right into their offices and personally tell them that you believe marijuana is good medicine and that you want them to support this bill when it comes to the floor. You already have some elected officials who are willing to put this bill to a vote, because they are aware of their constituents' wishes. So you don't have to *make* them do it, they are ready. They just need to know you support them.

"When you gather signatures to show your representative who in their district supports medical marijuana, I want you to redouble your efforts. I want you to get twice as many signatures, not because you need them, but because you want them. The problem is that your legislators are not hearing from you. You aren't hearing what you want to hear from them, but only because they haven't heard directly from you.

"Sixty percent. That's a lot of you. Ten years ago we couldn't get thirty percent. Ten years ago we got twenty percent, in one state. Now we have nine states using state legislation in violation of federal law.

"It is state law that matters to the citizens of the state. I think many of you would agree that you don't want the federal government in your doctor's office anymore, deciding what's best for you."

I pause and catch my breath, then hold up my closed can of marijuana. The shiny metal canister gleams in the sunlight. "I've been receiving this for about twelve years now. This can is a month's supply. It's full of marijuana and it comes all rolled. However, I don't plan to smoke a marijuana cigarette here in front of all of you today. That isn't relevant nor the reason I'm here.

"The purpose of this event is to let you know that you are in a wonderful position. You have both the legislators and the majority of the populace behind you. There is no better time to make known what the people want than right now."

I pull off the lid of the container, reach in, pull out a joint, and hold it up between my fingers. Members of the crowd surge forward and the sound of clicking cameras fills the air. It never fails. People are amazed and shocked at the site of the herb. As if being pulled in like a magnet, everyone moves closer.

"Every month I get three hundred of these joints from my doctor who gets them from the federal government." I put the joint back in the can and press on. "It is mostly leaf with some other parts of the plant mixed in. The government told us that we have to moisturize this to use it. So all the patients take the marijuana out of the cigarette paper it comes pre-rolled in, moisturize it, take the seeds and stems out of it and then re-roll and smoke it. Through this at-home processing, patients lose about twenty percent of what the government sends. However, that's how the federal government ensures that every joint is the same. Every time I smoke, I am getting the same dose of the same medicine. Compare that to what my doctors used to prescribe for me: three or four hundred morphine pills in a month. Nobody ever saw any problem with that.

"So we need to do a couple of things. We need to tell people that this issue is not about recreational smoking, it is about medicinal use. These patients need only their doctor's care. We don't need to mix the recreational argument into this issue, because it isn't relevant. These folks are *sick*. When you look at me and I am happy, does that mean I am high or does that mean I have some quality of life?"

I am interrupted by the shout of a reporter standing in the front of the crowd. "Could you hold that joint up again, the same way you did a few seconds ago?"

His request catches me off guard, but I shake my head and answer, "No, this isn't a side show."

The reporter says, "It's not like you are lighting it or anything."

I ignore his silly entreaty and press forward. "You already have your legislators at your side, but not all of them. You've still got some convincing to do, but you are doing it. Now, I'd be happy to take some informal questions from the audience."

The same reporter who interrupted me earlier lunges forward with a microphone and calls out in a loud voice, "Did the police ask you not to smoke here?"

This journalist does not bother to tell me his name or the publication for which he works. Although I find both that and his questions odd and unprofessional, I smile and even so, I am wary; I've been around long enough to know that despite ideals of fair and unbiased reporting, any journalist can skew the facts to fit his or her agenda and viewpoint. Sadly, it is my experience that politics infuses the majority of so-called objective information we receive from the mainstream press.

I figure I've got to give this reporter a chance, so I forgive his lack of decorum and move a little closer to him, so he won't have to shout any more questions. I shake my head and say, "No, the police didn't tell me that I couldn't smoke here. They *did* ask that I be mindful of my manners."

The reporter says, "The press release said that you would smoke dope on the capitol steps."

His choice of terminology irritates me somewhat and I say, "With all due respect, I don't smoke dope. I smoke cannabis. I don't know where you got that press release from, but it sure wasn't from me and I certainly never promised anyone else I was going to smoke at the capitol. It's not something I would normally do. Why would I step into a crowd of people and smoke pot?"

"Well, do you have a pass or something that proves it's legal for you to smoke?"

"No. Unfortunately, recipients of federally-produced medical marijuana have a terrible time trying to verify their status."

"So if these cops here wanted to bust you today, what is your argument against that? You have no paperwork, no nothing?"

"Sure, I've got lots of paperwork and I have the prescription labels on my can. Besides, I'm pretty well-known. I've been in lots of newspapers and magazines. But do I have official identification from the federal government? Absolutely not. They won't even admit I exist. If you contact the National Institute on Drug Abuse or the Drug Enforcement Administration, they will admit that there are patients who receive marijuana. The only thing the DEA is concerned with is making sure that I don't share my medicine with anybody, which I don't. But if the DEA admits they know who I am and where I am, then they have violated their protocol. They can't do that."

Before the reporter has a chance to interrogate me further, a few more people call out questions. After I answer them, a stocky, dark-skinned man with thick spectacles steps out of the crowd and says, "I want to extend an invitation for you to attend a brief meeting at the Arkansas Public Policy Project. We'd like to have you speak at an informal roundtable discussion."

I'm always cautious of involving myself with groups, *especially* groups I don't know anything about. Generally speaking, the bigger the group, the more infused it is with politics and hidden agendas. I don't want to find out the hard way I'm associating with a group that has an agenda counter to mine. "Well, I certainly appreciate the invitation, but I've never heard of your organization before."

"That's because we work behind the curtain, so to speak. We've been around for several decades since the civil rights movement. Some of our older members were involved in desegregating Central High School, and..."

"Wait a minute. Do you mean *the* Central High School?"

"That's the one. Have you heard about it?"

"Heard about it? I was a young boy when I saw the news footage of the black girl with the white dress, I can't remember her name..."

"Elizabeth Eckford."

"Right. It made me sick to my stomach to see that little girl being taunted and spit on by that hateful mob of racists gathered outside the school. I remember how proud I was to see her have so much courage in the face of that ignorance. What does your group do these days?"

"We're a committed group of local citizens whose purpose is to influence the policymaking process here at the capitol. We stimulate grassroots efforts and educate legislators on progressive issues. Our office is nearby, if you want to drop in. We would be honored to have you."

"The honor is all mine. Thank you, everyone, for coming today." The audience bursts into applause as I slowly descend the capitol steps. However, after talking to the man about Elizabeth Eckford, I'm oblivious to the crowd. I am in a state of total awe. I've got one foot in the past, the other foot in the future and my head in the here and now. It seems you can't make history without stepping back into it.

There was once a time in this country when the federal government took a stand for the constitutional rights of citizens, when confronted with state governments that tried to implement unconstitutional segregation policies. Now the states are taking the federal government to task for pushing unconstitutional policies that interfere with the rights of patients. If it isn't black citizens being protected from the states by the federal government, it's sick and dying people being protected from the federal government by the states. I'll be damned if the old adage isn't true. The more things change, the more they stay the same.

Politicians, like all people, are a mixed bag. Some are beholden to special interest lobbyists and for them, my very existence is a testimony to a truth they can't accept. When I first meet them, they often have stunned appearances on their faces, as if they are awakening from a long dream they thought was real.

As a rule, however, legislators are not my enemies. Some politicians are genuinely interested in the rights and needs of their constituents. I've had more than one take the time to listen and a few have actually risked their political skins by going to bat for me.

The rotten apples sure taste bad, though. A few crooked legislators have lied straight to my face, smiling at me in my presence, and then tried to take away my life behind closed doors. It's enough to make a guy question his faith in humanity.

I feel lucky to be a legal patient. I don't feel guilty about my status, but I can't take for granted what so many other patients need and lack. Nevertheless, my health depends on a steady supply of medicine. Since being accepted to the Compassionate IND Program, Uncle Sam has always come through eventually. I've never had any problems with the government scientists. When something needed to be fixed, they were responsive.

There have been occasions, however, when paperwork was lost, misinterpreted or rejected and the official process ground to a halt. This has delayed the shipment of my medicine for an extended period of time, sometimes weeks or months. Nobody wants to be held responsible for the medicine getting into the wrong hands, so my paperwork can be rejected anytime for any reason. They can send back the paperwork for something as minor as an un-dotted "i" or the letters being muddied by the photocopier.

There have been times that shipments were so delayed that I was forced to reduce my daily intake of cannabis in order to make my supply last. Every time this has happened it threw me into a state of discomfort, poor health and anxiety. As the pain, spasms and nausea grew worse, I was always confronted with the same dilemma. Should I break down and resort to smoking black market medicine?

I was sure I could find illegal marijuana if my life depended on it. I had many friends and family members who were willing to go through the dangerous process of purchasing it for me. Marijuana is everywhere—on the streets, in prisons, on college campuses and even schoolyards.

After giving it much thought, I reached the same conclusion every time. My state of health was important, but I wasn't going to let an insignificant bureaucrat make me break the law to obtain my medicine. Never again would I suffer the indignity of being treated like a criminal just because I wanted to live a semi-normal, less painful life. Even if this was being stubborn to the point of my own detriment, I didn't really feel like I had any other choice. I had to live, but I also had to live with myself.

I always toughed it out and called my federal and state senators and representatives. I even contacted the Food and Drug Administration several times to inquire about the status of my medicine. After being bounced around through a hierarchical network of anonymous voices, I could usually reach somebody who knew about the program and knew who I was.

Texas Senator Phil Gramm, a conservative Republican,

responded to my plea for assistance one time when my medicine was late. In his personal letter to me, he stated that although he did not agree that marijuana was medicine, he would fight to protect my legal rights as his constituent and as a resident of Texas. Fortunately, my medicine arrived and I never had to use his services, but I was grateful for his unwavering commitment to me in a time of great stress.

In October of 1991, I went to a university in northern Minnesota to hear a public debate between Edwin Meese III (former Attorney General under Ronald Reagan) and Gatewood Gailbraith (an activist, lawyer and former gubernatorial candidate). After the debate, Mr. Meese stepped into the mezzanine to visit with me for a few minutes. My wife and friends, Daryl Paulson (a cerebral palsy patient), and John Birrenbach (Director of the Institute of Hemp), were present at our conversation. Meese said that the government's anti-marijuana campaign went way too far and Americans have suffered for it.

I was absolutely flabbergasted to hear these words coming from the lips of a former Attorney General. I began to realize that even at the federal level, officials could be humble enough to learn and grow and admit their mistakes. It took courage for him to talk to me in public like that and I respected him for it.

That conversation changed my entire approach to reform. After talking with Edwin Meese, I didn't feel like I had to shout anymore. I figured that more people would listen if I whispered and I began to realize that even politicians agonized over issues and had consciences to which they must answer.

It's often hard to tell the difference between my friends and my enemies. To find an ally is always pleasant, but sometimes I find my nemesis in a close circle of associates. Some people who support medical marijuana with words fail to back it up with action. Some activists put their own egos above the needs of sick and dying people. Some supporters don't consider the potential ramifications of their impulsive actions. Still others are simply making too much money in the ever-lucrative black market to care at all about anyone but themselves.

Often my purported adversaries surprise me as well by

being staunch defenders of my rights. People like police officers, who provide security for my speaking engagements, state commissioners of public safety, who speak in support of medical marijuana, and heads of narcotics task forces, who are kind and compassionate. These people often tell me that they understand the difference between medicine and recreation, between patients and addicts.

When I go on a journey to speak with politicians, I don't like to bring activists along. I've seen too many instances where good bills were killed by the zealous propaganda of true believers who simply didn't have their facts right. It's a shame. They mean well and they have every right and responsibility to be involved in the process. However, they can do more harm than good. That is why I don't like to move in a group. I feel better operating on my own. When it's all said and done, I have no reason to hate anybody and I have many reasons to laud the members of all the organizations, from pro-marijuana groups to the state police.

5
Cannabis Cops, Unwarranted Stops

Sheriff John Brown always hated me,
For what, I don't know.
Every time I planted a seed
He said, "Kill it before it grows."
He said, "Kill them before they grow."

- Bob Marley

The Arkansas highway spreads out before us like a concrete welcome mat in the bright afternoon. Margaret holds steadfast to the wheel navigating through heavy highway traffic while I recline in the passenger seat.

Yesterday, after we left Little Rock, we drove through the town of Hope, the Arkansas birthplace of former President Bill Clinton. I was surprised and amused to learn the city named Hope is located in a county named Hempstead. It seems apropos.

It's been a long haul and we're dog-tired, but we've got many miles to go before we sleep. The tip of my joint lets off a fiery glow, illuminating my disfigured fingers, relieving my pain and lifting my spirits.

Christopher and the documentary film crew continue to follow us in their rental car. Christopher's scratchy voice calls to me over my hand-held radio. "You see that Motel 6 up ahead?"

I've traveled the highways of America so long that I barely notice those generic blue signs with giant red sixes on them. For me, they just fade into the passing scenery. I lift the radio to my mouth and, doing my best to imitate the voice of the motel chain's owner, Tom Bodet, I say, "Looks like they even left the light on for us!"

Christopher laughs. "Look right next to the motel; there's the Arkansas State Police Headquarters. I wonder if *they* left the light on for us."

I glance across Interstate 30 to see several geometric and bland government buildings with dozens of police vehicles parked out front. I chuckle and say, "Yeah, they probably did. Their lights are *always* on. I don't think we'll be checking in there, though."

I turn and look out my passenger window to see an elderly couple buzz by in a worn-out tank of a car. A man hunkers over the steering wheel, squinting at the road in front of him. A huge, upside-down American flag is painted on the side of the car. As they cruise ahead in the distance, my mind swirls with fear and hope.

Suddenly, Christopher begins shouting through my speaker, interrupting my thoughts. "George, quick! Look at the parking lot off to the right in front of that apartment complex! It's a police chase! Oh my God, do you see that?"

I gaze through the bug-splattered windshield, quickly scanning the lot. I see the rotating cherry and blueberry colored lights of four black and white cop cars chasing what appears to be an old beat-up Dodge. The five cars speed across the pavement, coming dangerously close to hitting several parked vehicles along the way. They finally jump the curb and race down a grassy hill, out of our field of vision.

It reminds me of one of those drug-bust scenes that play incessantly on nightly television "reality" shows like *COPS*, *America's Most Wanted*, *America's Wildest Police Chases* and *Stories of the Highway Patrol*. After a while all those damned chases look the same. I get numb watching them on the boob tube, but I've never had the opportunity to witness one firsthand.

"Man, Christopher! What's the likelihood of seeing something like that?"

"I don't know," he responds. "But it makes me kind of antsy, you know? I hope they don't decide to take their chase on the highway, because if they do, they'll be coming up right behind us. I don't need this kind of drama today."

I twist around to look out my rear window. It's difficult to see through the rush hour traffic, but the road behind us seems to be free of flashing lights and sirens for now. "There's nothing to worry about," I tell Christopher. "We're going to be fine. Those cops were probably just giving some driver a speeding ticket when he foolishly decided to run."

Christopher laughs and says, "It's close to the end of the month. You think they are trying to make their arrest quotas?"

"You never know. Then again, maybe they're taking a drunk driver off the road or catching a serial rapist. We can only hope."

I rarely get tense around law enforcement officials. After all, it's not like I'm doing anything illegal by smoking a joint. Besides, I grew up in a time when police were called upon to serve and protect, not control and incarcerate. And now, after September 11, police are being looked at again with respect even though some misguided legislators have tried to transform our peace officers into drug warriors to battle perpetrators who are really law abiding citizens in pain.

Though most officers are out on the streets trying to do their jobs and protect our lives, there is in any large group, a few renegade officers who act as though they are above the law. These are people who worship the raw power and arbitrary authority of the gun and the prison cell and who cannot distinguish between matters of public safety and individual liberty. A few of these officers have harassed and arrested friends of mine who were sick. One even physically assaulted me.

Christopher says, "You know, I'm pretty good friends with a deputy constable. We were talking the other day and he told me that he doesn't generally arrest people for smoking marijuana. He said that if he sees a joint in someone's car ashtray, he looks the other way, but if their kid is in the back seat without a seatbelt on, he'll ticket them."

"You might be surprised at how many officers will exercise their personal discretion when it comes to marijuana," I remark.

Christopher responds in agreement. "Yeah, I think most know they have bigger fish to fry. Even some county judges are refusing to lock people up for cannabis. They think it's a complete waste of taxpayer dollars."

"It makes sense if you think about it. There are plenty of child molesters and murderers who occupy or should occupy the immediate attention of law officials. Not to mention terrorists."

I drop the radio and take another toke from my joint. As we cruise the interstate arteries of the rural south, the sickly sweet scent of Arkansas evergreen trees drifts through the dashboard vent. I begin to reflect on all those faces behind the silver badges. After all is said and done, cops are just like the rest of us. Most are compassionate, some are ignorant and a few are just plain mean.

My first intimate experiences with law enforcement occurred before I was a legal marijuana patient, back when I had to rely on the black market for my medicine. In order to maintain my supply of marijuana, I was forced to make connections with some pretty shady people. Some of them even turned out to be undercover police officers in disguise.

One day a biker friend of mine, known among all the local folks as Dirty Bob, stopped by my house to see me. He pulled up in the front yard, riding a beautiful, shiny Harley-Davidson and dropped his bike unceremoniously down in the grass. He stepped into my house wearing a pair of Levi's so encrusted with dirt they matched his brown leather boots. He completed the outfit with a stained t-shirt under a leather vest and greasy hair that hung down to the middle of his back. He plopped down on the couch and I graciously offered him a joint.

He stayed quiet for a moment, then looked at me and said, "You don't know who I am, do you?"

I laughed and said, "Sure, you're Dirty Bob."

He shook his head and replied, "No, you don't know who I am." He rolled up his pant leg and pulled out a glistening badge. "I'm a police officer and I'm no longer undercover. Someone has been trying to bust you for the last two years and I really believe you deserve to know who I am."

I sat there with my illegal joint in hand, absolutely stunned. "Then why haven't you arrested me?"

"You've never been busted because you never did anything to warrant it. You never stole anything or bought stolen property.

You never sold drugs. You never hurt anybody. All you did was smoke pot. I've known you for a couple of years and I think I know you pretty well."

I was in a state of complete bewilderment. I couldn't believe what he was telling me. I had always felt I was savvy enough to be a fairly accurate judge of people. Usually I had no reason to take people for anything other than who they said they were.

I'd seen this guy at all times of the day and night and I knew what kind of people he hung out with. There were no alarms going off in my head that would have made me suspect this guy was a police officer. Dumbfounded, I finally managed to say, "Yeah, you know me."

Dirty Bob grinned and said, "I'm one of the top narcotics agents in this state. I'm good at what I do. Most people never see it coming. And I'm one of the best at catching people trying to fence stolen property to get drugs. I hate thieves."

I looked him straight in the eyes. "I understand."

He pointed at me. "If you ever have any trouble with the police, you tell them to call me. Okay? I will vouch for your character."

"Sure. Thanks, Bob."

He stood up and strode out of my house almost as quickly and unassumingly as he had entered. I kicked back on the couch and lit a joint as I heard the explosive, guttural belch of his bike taking off down my driveway.

Dirty Bob was a good undercover cop, one of the best. I never would have guessed his occupation if he hadn't shared it with me. As I sat there smoking my joint, I had no idea that his calling card would save me someday.

One day I got a phone call from a man who was trying to sell a Harley-Davidson motorcycle and said a mutual friend had suggested he contact me. He asked if I would be interested in buying it. I told him I might, but I needed to see it first. He invited me to stop by his home the next night so I could check out the bike. He gave me directions and said, "When you arrive, just come to the back door and let yourself in. I may still have some associates over for a meeting, but if you don't mind waiting a few minutes, I'll be happy to show you the bike."

The next day, Margaret and I went to the man's house at the appointed time. We parked on the street and walked up to the back door of the house.

As soon as we stepped inside, I had a weird feeling in the pit of my stomach, like an alarm. The place was dark. The only light we could see came from a room down a hallway. Blowing off the wary feeling in my gut, I walked cautiously through the back of the house toward the one lit room with Margaret following close behind.

When I pushed the door open, eight strangers lounging around a coffee table turned and stared. Apparently, we stumbled upon the as yet unfinished meeting. Margaret and I stood awkwardly in the doorway for a moment as sixteen eyes looked us over. I had never met him, so I assumed the owner of the motorcycle I had come to look at was one of the eight men. Not wanting to interrupt his meeting, I muttered, "Sorry for the intrusion. We can just wait until you're finished." I pulled Margaret over to two empty chairs and we quietly sat down. The men resumed their discussion, but before long, some of the guys started talking about drugs. That was it for me. Standing up, I said, "I don't want to hear about any of this. We'll wait in another room. Come on, Margaret." We got up and walked out of the room.

We sat down in the darkened dining room for a few minutes debating whether or not we should just leave. Finally, we decided to go back to the group to tell the bike's owner that we'd come back another time. When we walked back to the bedroom and pushed open the door, we got the shock of our lives: two of the men were pointing guns in our direction. One of them held a .357-caliber, nickel-plated, six-shooter revolver aimed straight at my face. As if that wasn't enough to make me nervous, I could see that his hands were trembling. I felt like I was going to be sick.

The man with the .357 shouted, "GET ON YOUR FACE! NOW! GET DOWN! GET DOWN! GET DOWN!"

Margaret and I immediately dropped to the floor. Lying there, my wife begged, "Please, whatever reason you think we're here for, we're not. We just came here to look at a Harley."

I too didn't want to make a bad situation worse by mouthing

off or arguing. "Hey, whatever you say, man. Look, we don't want any trouble. If it's money you want, I have some in my wallet. Take it, it's yours."

The man with the jittery grip yelled back, "I'M A COP!"

Surprised but a little relieved that we weren't dealing with thugs, I looked up slowly and asked, "May I see your badge?"

"Don't move!" he said sternly as he released one trembling hand from his gun and reached for his badge. The gun stopped shaking quite so violently which made me feel a little safer.

Just then, there were three quick, loud knocks at the front and back doors. Then I heard a muffled voice shout, "OPEN UP! WARRANT!" Suddenly, the doors burst open and five police officers, all dressed in plainclothes with black jackets and big guns, came running into the house.

Apparently, the owner of the bike had also been selling drugs to local kids and the police had been staking out his home for quite some time. I'd just unknowingly walked into the middle of a narcotics bust. My timing was impeccable.

The police turned on lights all over the house and brought me and Margaret into another room to begin their first round of intensive questioning. They wanted me to tell them everything I knew about the illegal activities taking place at this house.

I knew nothing, of course. I looked right in the eyes of the officer who had pulled the gun on me and said, "I don't know what's going on here. This guy is a friend of a friend. I don't even know him personally. He called me about a bike he is selling. You saw me leave the room when everyone started talking about drugs. I don't want anything to do with that nonsense. I just came here to look at a Harley-Davidson for sale."

The officer admitted to the other interrogators and his superior, who eyed me skeptically, that what I'd said about leaving the room was true. Yet it was obvious that they weren't buying my story and were seconds away from cuffing me and hauling me off to the slammer.

That was when Margaret began to lose her temper. My wife is generally a soft-spoken woman, but when she thinks her family is being attacked, she comes out fighting like a lioness protecting her cubs. She started yelling at the officers. "Why are you threatening my husband? He didn't do anything! He wasn't even in the room! Why are you giving him a hard time?"

My mind raced. Surely there was a way out of this. Suddenly, I remembered what Dirty Bob told me. "Hey! I know just the person you need to talk to. Get Lieutenant Bob on the phone. He's one of the top narcotics officers in the police department and he knows I'm not a drug dealer. He'll tell you what kind of guy I am."

The officers looked surprised when I mentioned him and one of them asked, "How do you know Bob? Have you been busted before?"

"No, it's not like that. Just call him."

"Okay," one of the officers said. "I guess we better check this out. We'll get Bob on the line, but if we find out you are lying to us, then you just made things that much harder on yourself." He walked across the room to the telephone and dialed while another officer watched me sweat.

I contemplated the situation. It was late in the evening. Was Dirty Bob even at home? Or could he have turned in early and be sound asleep? In that case, would he hear the telephone ring? I looked over at the officer on the telephone. His lips began moving. *Aha, he's gotten through to somebody!* I felt a little better, but I could-n't hear what was being said. As the seconds turned to minutes, I became increasingly nervous. *What if Bob couldn't or wouldn't vouch for me after all?* My heart was pounding. It was a very tense five minutes.

The cop hung up the phone and slowly walked back over to me with a blank, business-like expression on his face. "You are free to go, Mr. McMahon. Don't come back here and don't ever let us see you at any drug dealer's house again."

I was relieved but flabbergasted. How was I supposed to know the guy was a drug dealer? I came to that house to buy a bike and I left there with a bunch of cops treating me like a criminal who was just lucky enough to get a last-minute "get out of jail free" pass. *Still, it could have been much worse,* I told myself. I resisted the urge to argue with the cop and quickly left the house, thankful the whole affair was over.

My days of illegally smoking pot for alleviation of my pain are long gone. Federal law now allows me to smoke cannabis in any public place. As for private property I can smoke anywhere as long as I have the consent of the owner.

I've always tried to be considerate of other people's concerns. Even though I am legally allowed to smoke cannabis in public areas where cigarette smoking is prohibited, I never do this, because I have no wish to offend anyone. I also never smoke in public places where children tend to congregate, like school playgrounds or public parks. That would only serve to entrench the already prevalent, irrational anxieties associated with marijuana. Furthermore, I don't want to encounter and have to assuage the fears of frightened parents or argue with teachers, administrators and police. If I know I'm going to be in a public place for an extended period of time and will need to smoke, such as appearing before a legislature, attending a conference or speaking at a high school forum, I always inform the proper authorities ahead of time. We then discuss and agree upon a plan that meets their needs and my own. This protects everybody's interests and has always worked for me.

I've smoked marijuana in many strange places over the years and most bystanders have shown me basic respect and courtesy. I think that in spite of dirty politics, tolerance still thrives in the hearts of most Americans. Even when I smoked pot on Pennsylvania Avenue in Washington, D.C., right in front of the White House, nobody called the police on me.

One time I smoked marijuana under the dome of the United States capitol building. Margaret and I had traveled to the District of Columbia so we could talk to federal legislators about medical marijuana. At the time, I had a relapse and was in a wheelchair, but I stubbornly refused to stay in it. Instead, I rolled all the way up to the front door of each congressman's office, then I stood up and walked in using a cane.

Although I was technically allowed to smoke pot inside the building, I really didn't want to deal with explaining my legal status to the police. However, after a long day, I was worn out and in pain;

I needed my medicine. So I decided to take a very quick puff under the capitol dome. Discreetly lighting my joint, I took a drag and snubbed it out on my fingertip as I sat in my wheelchair, right next to a looming statue of Thomas Jefferson. That prophetic founding forefather once wrote that *cannabis sativa* was "of first necessity to the wealth and protection of the country." I wish he had written "health" instead of "wealth."

A few years later I was driving through a small town in north Texas, on the final leg of an exhausting thirty-hour drive from Washington, D.C., where I had spoken at a medical marijuana conference. A friend had driven the majority of the way, but there were seven hours between his house, where I dropped him off, and mine.

I was still over an hour from home when I realized I was too tired to be behind the wheel. Not wanting to take any chances, I pulled off to the side of the road and slept for twenty minutes. After I woke up and began driving again, it soon became clear the twenty minute nap wasn't quite enough to fully recuperate. Instead of getting on the highway, I wound up taking a wrong turn on a loop that sent me back toward the small Texas town I had just driven through. As I noticed signs telling me that I was going the wrong way, a police cruiser pulled up behind me and its lights began flashing. We both pulled over and the officer got out of his vehicle.

He walked cautiously up to my car, then asked me who I was and where I was going. I gave the officer my name and told him I was coming from Washington, D.C., but he kept asking me the same questions over and over again. "Where have you been? Where are you going? How long have you been driving? How long have you been awake? How are you feeling? Did you know that you were headed into town?" He was courteous and respectful throughout the course of his questioning and I could tell that he was worried about my safety. The officer told me I needed to pull over and rest some more before I went any further.

I told him that I was driving home from a medical marijuana conference. After a short pause he said, "You don't happen to have any of that medical marijuana with you, do you?"

I looked straight into his wary eyes and said, "As a matter of fact, I never go anywhere without it."

His mouth dropped open and his eyes opened wide like he had just gotten the shock of his life. Yet he wasn't mad or suspicious, just very surprised. He sputtered, "Really? And it's legal?"

"I'm one of the legal marijuana patients approved by the federal government."

The officer wore an expression of amazement. "I've heard of that before, but do you have anything on you that will prove that?"

I reached for my briefcase, got out of the truck and walked around to the back so I could give him my paperwork showing that I was a recipient of government marijuana.

The papers rustled in his hands as the wind blew. "Holy cow," he exclaimed, "I've never seen anything like this! You realize I'm going to have to call this in and check on it."

I told him that he could contact the Washington bureau of the Drug Enforcement Agency or the Texas Rangers at the state capitol in Austin.

The officer hesitated and then asked, "Can I see the marijuana?"

"Sure, but it's up front, in my suitcase in the cab of my truck." We returned to the front of the truck and I set my briefcase in the passenger seat.

The officer pointed and said, "Is that some of the medical marijuana on the floor of your truck?"

I looked down and tried not to laugh. "No, sir. That's just yard grass and tobacco from the trip. You don't want to search my truck, do you?"

"No, I don't think that will be necessary."

I pulled out the big silver canister from my suitcase and handed it to the officer. He stared at the prescription label on the lid of the can. He didn't open the container, but he held it up to his nose and sniffed it.

"That sure does smell like marijuana."

I nodded patiently. "Yep. That's what's in there."

After handing my canister back to me, he sauntered towards his squad car, then turned and said, "You don't have to stand outside while I call this in, Mr. McMahon. You can sit in your truck if you want." He didn't even make me take my keys out of the ignition or shut off my engine.

The officer sat in his car a few minutes trying to verify my story. Finally, after he got in touch with an official who confirmed that I was free to leave with my marijuana, he again approached my truck.

"Well, Mr. McMahon, I've verified your story. I have to say, it's really amazing. I never would have believed it. Listen, I've got kind of a special request. If you don't mind, could I actually *see* your marijuana?"

I opened the can for him and let him look at my government joints. He shook his head in astonishment, thanked me and then drove off in his squad car, hopefully to catch some real criminals. I bet he told his buddies about me when he got back to the station.

What was notable to me about the experience was that I never once felt threatened. The officer was professional and courteous throughout the entire interrogation. He treated me decently and so I felt comfortable talking to him honestly. There was no negative attitude or ulterior motives.

After I got home, the story of my traffic stop made its way through the grapevine to a friend who knew the officer who stopped me. He called to tell me that officer was in charge of the local K-9 drug unit. I hoped the officer learned something about medical marijuana the day he met me.

However, not all Texas officers have been so accommodating. One time my wife and I were at the state capitol building in Austin. We wanted to talk to our state representatives about a medical marijuana bill that was pending in the Criminal Jurisprudence Committee.

When Margaret and I arrived, we let the capitol security guards know who we were and that we were there to talk to several senators. As we walked through the capitol building, I suddenly noticed an endless number of police officers trying to subtly keep their eyes on me. They seemed to come out of the woodwork, doors and hallways and they were absurdly obvious, barely making an effort to be discreet. When I stepped onto an elevator, a ranger that had been tailing me followed me right in. Then, when I decided the elevator was too crowded and stepped out, the ranger did the same and stood next to me as I waited for the next elevator to arrive.

On the one hand, I understood why the capitol police in Austin were so nervous. In all fairness, my associates neglected to tell them I was coming. However, their actions bordered on the ridiculous and I didn't like what I viewed as their efforts at intimidation.

After speaking with the first senator on my contact list, I stepped out into the hallway that led toward the main senate chamber, a huge solemn room where a relatively small group of politicians decide who will pay, who will profit and who will go to jail.

Six capitol police officers were waiting for me in the chamber and they didn't hesitate to approach me directly. One big guy who was obviously in charge, said, "Mr. McMahon, can you show me a driver's license or some identification that proves who you are?"

"I don't have a driver's license," I said, pulling out my Oakland Cannabis Buyers' Club card. I had picked it up while I was in California. I handed it to him and asked, "Will this do?"

He said, "Yeah, this will be fine. I already phoned the Drug Enforcement Administration. I just needed to verify your identity. Have a good day, Mr. McMahon."

Later, my wife and I noticed that a plainclothes policeman followed us everywhere we went in the capitol building. He even walked behind us through the front doors as we were leaving the building. As we walked away, he stood on the capitol steps watching us go like a relieved babysitter, anxious to see that we were really leaving the property.

Ten years earlier, the scene would have bothered me and insulted my sense of dignity. Then again, most people treated me with respect even back in the early days of my legal use. For example, shortly after I became a Compassionate IND patient, I planned a visit to the Iowa State Capitol in Des Moines. The state police took the time to write a letter notifying me that if the weather was bad, if it should rain or even if I didn't feel well, I would have a designated indoor area in which I could smoke.

Nowadays, I don't get too angry when officers do what they think is their job, so long as they know what their job is. And most of them *do* know. They know I'm not a danger or a menace. I may threaten some of the political myths they believe in, but they know I pose no immediate threat to public safety.

Officers who are truly just doing their job will keep their personal opinions out of the legal equation. They simply follow the rules and act professionally, leaving no room for personal beliefs. It doesn't matter to the true professionals how much they hate me or what I stand for, so long as I am not breaking the law. I don't have to worry too much, once they know I'm legal. Then they quickly get the message and act to preserve my rights.

Whenever I've returned to the capitol building in Austin since that day, I feel very comfortable. I haven't noticed anybody following me. I don't call to tell them I'm coming. I just show up.

I have the feeling they already know who I am.

However, my forty-seventh birthday was nearly spoiled by an overzealous police officer. It was 1997, a year after California led the state reform movement by removing criminal penalties for qualifying patients who used, possessed, or grew medical mari- juana. Proposition 215 was approved by California voters on November 5, 1996. Despite public sentiment in California and many other states, in Texas, that feeling was not shared, especially not by law enforcement.

Some of my friends took me out to celebrate my birthday. They rented a fully equipped, ten-passenger, slick white limousine. Margaret and I seldom got the chance to sit in a limo, so it was a big thrill.

We filled up the limo and started a tour of town, driving down an opulent street the locals referred to as "millionaire row." After seeing how the other half lives, my friends suggested going to a casino on a nearby Indian reservation.

I've never been much of a gambling man. Maybe it's because I never had enough cash in my pocket to justify taking a chance on pissing it away. Or perhaps my daily life of sickness and surgery already held enough risks.

I said, "I don't gamble."

I turned to my wife who said, "I don't gamble, either."

My friend, Henry, shrugged and said, "Well, we could still go there and have a nice dinner. If we end up staying a couple of hours, the casino will probably pay for our meals."

Henry's wife, Diana, had a fever for the crap tables and I had to admit I was terribly hungry. Finally, I said, "Alright, sounds great. Let's go."

We drove to the casino and immediately went to the restaurant to eat. After waiting two full hours to be served, we found the food was really terrible. It was so bad, I felt ill after I ate it. I got up and left the table in disgust.

Over the next hour Margaret and I spent a grand total of about five dollars on the slot machines. At that point, we had been in the casino for three hours. Annoyed and bored, Margaret and I walked around while our friends gambled, mesmerized by the flashing lights and ringing bells. We were more than ready to leave, but my buddies were winning big and wanted to stay a while longer.

Tired of the casino, I left and walked across the parking lot to the limousine. Climbing into the plush vehicle, I pulled out a joint and lit it. I hadn't smoked for hours and was in enough pain to need some medicine.

A few minutes later, the driver got in the front seat of the limo and told me that my friends were ready to go. We drove up to the front of the casino to pick up our motley crew. One guy in our group had just won more than $1500 and another had won $700. They were anxious to take the money and run. I was just relieved to be heading home.

Suddenly, before we pulled away from the curb, a parking lot attendant ran up to our car and said angrily "I know you people are out here smoking marijuana. I know the smell of pot!"

I turned and asked Henry, "You want me to get out and tell

this guy who I am?"

He said, "Well, it might help."

I climbed out and said to the security attendant, "Look, I'm not trying to cause any problems. I'm one of the federal marijuana patients. I did go out to the car alone to smoke a joint to ease my pain as required by my legal prescription."

The attendant looked at me like I was either lying, psychotic or both. "Wait right here," he said sternly and ran back inside the casino.

Not wanting to make a scene or be chased by police, we stayed put. After a few brief moments the attendant came back outside, stood right in front of the limo, and shouted with an exaggerated sense of authority, "You need to wait here! I've called casino security and they're on their way."

The air was thick, humid and hot, but we all waited in silence until the casino security officer showed up. When he did, I pulled out a flyer announcing a speech I was giving on medical cannabis and my medicine bottle with a prescription label on it.

The security officer said, "Don't bother giving me excuses. I've already called the county sheriff and they are coming to get you."

We waited and waited. Finally fed up, I said, "This is ridiculous. We can clear this up right here and now. I've already shown you my prescription bottle and a flyer that says who I am and what I'm doing."

The security officer shook his head, pointed his finger at me and said, "I don't care what you show me. I don't even care if God himself walks in here and tells me that you are a legal federal marijuana patient. I still want to see you get arrested."

"So no proof I offer will prevent you from turning this into a bad scene."

He said, "None."

Now I started to get really angry. The tension was rising. My buddies paced in circles, growing madder by the second.

Finally, after forty minutes of waiting, the county sheriff pulled into the parking lot and jumped out of his squad car. He looked me over and said, "Please hand over that prescription and come with me."

"Are you arresting me?"

"No. I'd just like you to come with me to department head-quarters so we can get this cleared up."

Feeling I had no other option, I followed the sheriff and climbed into the backseat of his vehicle. He drove me to the local police department with my friends and wife following close behind in the limo.

As I followed the sheriff through the back door of the police station, I felt like I was trapped in an absurd episode of *Gun Smoke*.

The deputy sheriff pointed to a chair and said, "I'm not going to lock you up, okay? You can sit down out here and wait a few minutes while I verify what's going on here."

"No problem." I was annoyed at the inconvenience but was not too distressed by the events. In fact, I've learned to expect them occasionally. I sat down on the bench, sighing with resignation.

The sheriff placed my prescription bottle on the front counter. Then he turned to me and asked, "What's the phone number of your local sheriff?"

I couldn't believe he expected me to know this information off the top of my head. "I'm sorry, sir, but I don't know. I don't exactly have the number memorized."

The sheriff left me sitting there while he searched for the number in his files. I looked at my prescription bottle. According to federal law, if I had needed to, I could have stepped outside for a joint. The clerk at the front desk of the station kept glancing at me like I had just arrived to earth from another planet.

About fifteen minutes later, the sheriff emerged from the back of the police station, sauntered into the lobby and handed my container of marijuana to me. "I was finally able to clear it up. Your local law enforcement officials vouched for you."

"Just like I knew they would."

"I'm sorry if I offended you. I don't see this sort of thing everyday and it was the only way I knew to handle it."

"I understand."

As I walked toward the exit I felt vindicated, but I couldn't get the bad taste of the scene out of my mouth. A beautiful birthday evening was ruined by one overzealous security guard's insatiable desire to give somebody trouble. I don't know what his problem was, but it was hard to believe that someone could be that obstinate without a serious reason.

The limo driver called a few days later to tell me the casino operator had contacted the director of the limousine company asking them to pass along a message to me. They offered to supply me with a smoking room if I ever returned. They didn't call it an "apology." They called it a "compensation" for the unnecessary trouble. Needless to say, I've never been back.

Christopher's voice over the handheld radio interrupts my thoughts of the past.

"See that diner up ahead? Let's stop. I'm starving."

I look over at Margaret who nods. "Sounds good," I answer.

We pull into the diner parking lot and climb out of our cars. Though everyone is hungry, no one really feels like sitting right away. We stretch and talk in the parking lot for a few minutes before finally heading inside for a meal.

After we are seated and order our food, a documentary crew member asks to hear one of my many stories of "close encounters" with the police.

"Yeah, tell them about the assault in Virginia," Christopher says with a grin. He's already heard most of these stories but for some reason, he never tires of hearing them again.

"Well," I begin, "It was the summer of 1995. Margaret and I were invited to attend a three-day conference sponsored by the National Institute of Drug Abuse. The speaking itinerary included psychologists and psychiatrists who were disseminating false information about how marijuana was dangerous and physically addictive. I felt it was my duty to prove they were wrong."

Christopher chuckles. "Sounds like the George I know."

I continue. "These so-called experts came up with all these anecdotal accounts, but they offered no evidence, because, as you all know, there is none. Marijuana doesn't affect the addiction centers of the brain."

The waitress comes by to pour our coffee. I point to the cups. "At worst, marijuana is a habit like drinking coffee or eating candy. You don't *need* the caffeine or the sugar, but they sure do make you feel energized.

"Anyway, it was tough for Margaret and me to attend, both financially and physically, but we were determined to appear so we could dispute the misguided 'experts.' The conference was located right where the three corners of Virginia, Maryland and the District of Columbia come together. There's lots of towering hotels linked by underground temperature controlled walkways so people don't have to go outside in the cold winter weather or, in our case, the intense summer heat. As a result, there wasn't much in the way of public transportation or taxicabs available so we were forced to walk everywhere we needed to go.

"While this arrangement is fine for healthy people, it was hard on Margaret and me. You all know how my energy gets depleted when I move a lot. Plus, I didn't take a wheelchair on this trip, so I was on foot. By the time we got up to our room, we were about a half-mile from where the conference was actually meeting and we were both exhausted.

"The first day of the conference was a long one. I left early and asked a security officer if he knew of a good place where I could smoke. He directed me to a private stairwell open to the outdoors. Hotel guests were welcome to travel on the stairs, but not many did."

I pause as the waitress serves our meals. Then, as the others begin eating, I go on. "On the third evening of the conference, Margaret and I sat on the steps and talked with a marijuana activist who worked for a hemp clothing company. We were sitting on the steps where I discreetly smoked my medicine, when all of a sudden two men emerged from a nearby crowd of conference attendees and headed our way. One of them was the security officer who had designated this area for us to smoke in. He was accompanied by a tall, well-built man wearing a football jacket. At first I thought the guy in the jacket was somebody NIDA officials didn't want at the conference, since it appeared that he was being escorted away by the security officer. When they passed us, he gave me a really dirty look. I was relieved when they walked right by us.

"Suddenly, the two men turned around and came at us. The security guard began yelling, 'Put that out! Put that out!' Then he flicked the end of my joint with his fingers, trying to knock the glowing tip from the cigarette. I was totally baffled by this bizarre behavior and I instinctively pulled my hands away.

"Then the guy in the football jacket stepped between Margaret and me. He slapped my hand hard, knocking the joint to the ground. I cried out in pain. The bones in my hand are so brittle that he could have easily broken one of my fingers or my wrist.

"Both men were standing over Margaret and me, trying to intimidate us with their physical presence. Our activist friend sat in stunned silence, his mouth gaping wide in complete disbelief. The guys ignored him. They obviously were after me and me alone."

"Holy shit! What did you do, George?" the documentary cameraman asks.

"Well, being in the shape I'm in, I can't start a physical fight with anyone. But I was mad as hell. I looked at the two thugs and said, 'What the hell is wrong with you?'

"Poor Margaret was trembling with fear and anger, but she bravely stood up and shouted, 'He's legal! Leave him alone!'"

"You just don't mess with Margaret," Christopher says with a smile.

"I wanted to kick his ass," Margaret replies. "Wait until you hear what happened next."

I lower my voice. "I don't want the whole restaurant to hear this. The guy in the leather jacket looked at my wife and wagged his finger in her face screaming, 'You shut your fucking mouth! You hear me, you mother-fucking bitch?'"

"Whoa! That's insane. What a psycho," the cameraman says.

"And it didn't stop there," I explain. "The guy continued assaulting us with vile names as he kept hitting my hands and wrists. God, what I wouldn't have done to be healthy and strong for just one moment so I could have stood up and kicked that guy's ass. It's one thing to be disrespectful to me. It's quite another to talk that way to Margaret. But what could I do? I was a sick man with a cane and this guy was built like a bear and clearly had a temper to match.

"Margaret and I were totally defenseless against them. At that moment I thought that anything could happen and I truly feared for our lives. For all I knew, this wacko was going to pull out a gun and shoot us.

"Not knowing what else to do, I asked again, 'What's wrong with you? If you don't leave me alone, I'm going to call the cops!'

"That's when this son-of-a-bitch bent down and put his sneering lips right next to my ear and whispered, 'I'm a Virginia narcotics officer, motherfucker! Don't smoke here again, you bastard!'"

"Oh my God," a documentary crewmember says. "What happened next?"

"Luckily, both men turned and quickly disappeared into the secure anonymity of the crowd."

"That's absolutely crazy, George."

"Yeah. Unfortunately, there's all kinds of jerks in this world and some of them just happen to be police officers. I've been bullied before, but I had never experienced anything even close to what happened that time. I mean, this guy was more a gangster than a cop.

"After that incident, Margaret and I were quite shaken and decided to head right to our hotel room where we would feel safe. As we walked through the lobby, I became angrier and angrier thinking about what happened. I decided I wasn't going to just sit back and take it, so I began to make phone calls as soon as we walked into our room. Several attorneys at the conference offered their generous assistance and before it was over, officials woke up a Virginia Superior Court judge at two o'clock in the morning so he could resolve the issue. He ruled that since I was accepted into the IND Program, I had the legal right to smoke marijuana anywhere, including inside the conference area if I chose to."

"Sometimes justice prevails," Christopher says, grabbing

the bill our waitress has just dropped on the table.

"Yeah, but it was a bitter victory in a senseless battle. I was hurting nobody by taking my medicine at a government-sponsored conference where my dignity and safety should have been assured. Instead an undercover narcotics officer decided to play John Wayne with my constitutional rights."

We all put in money for the bill, hit the bathrooms and head out to our cars to continue our journey. As I sit back in the passenger seat beside Margaret, I think about how tough a handful of cops have made my life over the years. Although I'm a legal marijuana smoker, if a cop really wants to, he could legally arrest me and hold me in a cell, separated from my medicine for several days, while he takes his sweet time verifying my identity and legal status. By the time the cell door is unlocked, my health could be compromised to the point where I'd need immediate medical attention.

I'm sure I could win a lawsuit if an officer ever tried anything like that, but the promise of future compensation holds little value for a man when he's sick and dying. I would rather just live in peace and, thankfully, I've been able to do that for the most part.

Not every patient has been so lucky. Many languish in prison for their use of black market marijuana. Others were forced to stop using medical marijuana and died because of it. Until all patients are able to receive the medicine they so desperately need, I will not stop speaking out, traveling the country and fighting for this precious cause.

⫼ 6
Pot Peers

Tell me how much you know of the sufferings of your fellow men and I will tell how much you have loved them.

– Helmut Thielicke

I open my eyes to see Elvis Presley staring down from the portrait that hangs on the bedroom wall. He looms over me like Frankenstein's monster revived from the netherworld. His upper lip is twisted into a permanent sneer and he seems to mock me as I rise from the king-size bed. I try to rub the sleep from my eyes and realize that I'm not dreaming. I'm at the Heartbreak Hotel in Memphis, Tennessee. It's down at the end of Lonely Street, literally. I saw the street sign.

I grab the remote control from the nightstand and switch on the television to hear the local weather report. Instead of the news, the television starts blaring "Rock-A-Hula-Baby" as Elvis shimmies on the screen, draped in a Hawaiian flower shirt. I try to mute it, but the music jolts Margaret awake beside me. I can't believe it: a twenty-four hour Elvis channel.

Before we departed on this journey, I tried to make Christopher understand. It's true that I grew up listening to Elvis like everyone my age did and I even really liked some of his songs, but I never considered him to be a hero or a demigod. To me, he was just another man, no better or worse than anyone else and all the hoopla surrounding his life and death is offensive to me.

My heroes are ordinary folks: manual laborers who know what it feels like to hurt at the end of a long day, aides who provide care for elderly patients in nursing homes, union members who are willing to fight for their causes, parents struggling to raise decent children in a violent, chaotic world and common folks who know the value of true friendship. These are the people I grew up admiring and wanting to emulate and I continue to hold them in esteem today.

Margaret and I shuffle drowsily around the room, preparing for the long day ahead. Our hotel quarters are fit for a king, no pun intended. After a shower and shave, I smoke my medicine. Then we head for the downstairs waiting area, which is filled with gaudy retro furniture, reminiscent of the fabulous fifties.

Leaning against the registration counter, the concierge waves to my wife and me as we step across the plush velvety carpet that skirts the hotel lobby. The managers and employees at the Heartbreak Hotel have been extremely courteous and accommodating. They were made aware of my medical and legal status before we arrived and yet they haven't insisted on seeing my paperwork. They ensured that my suite was reserved on the smoking floor, right next to an industrial strength smoke-eater, so other hotel patrons and security staff won't become alarmed at the smell of marijuana wafting down the halls. To top it off, they've given me two free passes for Graceland, including the mansion, the Lisa Marie airplane tour, the automobile museum and the Sincerely Elvis museum. I never expected such royal treatment and I'm grateful for the unsolicited hospitality.

As Margaret and I make our way through the front doors of the hotel and emerge in the brilliant morning sunlight, hidden loudspeakers blare the classic Presley standard, "Big Ole Hunk of Love." My head is splitting as we walk toward Graceland proper.

We arrive to find Christopher sitting at a table outside the visitor's center, chewing the last gooey bite of a deep-fried-in-butter peanut butter and banana sandwich, just like the ones Elvis used to gorge on. My wife sits down next to him and gazes at the graffiti-covered wall that encircles the Graceland mansion.

Unlike me, Margaret and Christopher are absolutely wild about Elvis. Although Christopher might never admit that publicly. When I first asked him if he liked Elvis, he tried to feed me some academic line of crap about iconography and cultural archetypes. He didn't fool me, though. I knew better, because I had seen the inside of Christopher's apartment. He's got pictures of Elvis hanging all over the walls, two Elvis clocks, Elvis mugs, an Elvis calendar and an Elvis T-shirt. The crowning glory of his gaudy collection is a plaster bust of the King of Rock and Roll. The stark white, disembodied head hovers above his refrigerator, like something in a morbid museum showcase.

Christopher stands up reverently, his long black hair blowing in the wind as he surveys the royal palace from afar. He turns to me and asks, "You know why we had to come here, George?"

"Yeah," I say with smirk. "Because you and my wife have totally gone off the deep end and you believe the reincarnated Elvis lives inside of you."

"That's close, but no cigar."

To counter his point, I reach in my pocket, pull out a cigarette and light it. A tram filled with starry-eyed tourists passes through the famous "music notes" front gate. I grin as I exhale the smoke.

"Seriously, George. Think about it. Elvis was addicted to painkillers, barbiturates and amphetamines during the final years of his life. Even though he was slowly killing himself, he didn't really think of himself as a drug addict. After all, the 'medication' he took was obtained legally, prescribed through his government-licensed doctor. These pills weren't the same as 'drugs.' Elvis hated illegal substances, including marijuana. He was so anti-drug he even showed up at the White House one day asking for a police badge from the Federal Bureau of Narcotics and he wrote President Nixon a letter about how illegal drugs and hippie counterculture were destroying society."

"That sounds like a man in some serious denial," I say. "He was probably high on amphetamines when he met Nixon. You know he took prescription speed as well as sleep and pain medications, right?"

Margaret chimes in, "Yeah, but it was the *legal* stuff that killed him."

I reply, "Not the drugs themselves, of course, but the way he used them."

It amuses me that people come from around the globe to gaze at this place. They call it hallowed ground. A few fanatical devotees have literally moved halfway across the world, just so they can live close to the mansion. I once heard that Graceland receives more annual visitors than the White House.

I look around the crowded outdoor mall, trying to decide if it is a dream or a nightmare. A mentally retarded man with an enormous grin who appears to suffer from Down's Syndrome, paces up and down the walkway, wiggling his fingers as he rocks back and forth humming "Love Me Tender." He is clad in full Elvis regalia, including dark sunglasses and a silver jumpsuit. He wears a long white cape with sparkling, ruby-red jewels affixed to the cloth. There's something I like about this guy. He seems so happy in spite of his disability. I consider saying hello to him, but I don't want to ruin his moment of glory.

I'm amazed at how many sick people I see around me. A Graceland employee assists a frail, elderly woman to a nearby bench. A bearded man with no legs rolls by in a wheelchair. A young boy with a shaved head and the telling pallor of recent chemotherapy holds hands with a man wearing a T-shirt from the Make-A-Wish Foundation.

There's something distinctly American about this eclectic collage of ailing humanity. They seem to blend in naturally with the swarming crowd of healthy tourists from all over the world. There is no prolonged staring, whispered mockery or condescending sympathy from the people here. There's no need for that sort of thing at Graceland. After all, in a way, when you come here, everyone is a freak.

I'm beginning to feel at home here, in a strange kind of way, and I can finally say that I'm glad we came. I'm too tired to take the full tour, but Christopher has graciously agreed to escort Margaret through the mansion while I wait in the courtyard.

After I finish my smoke, my wife and Christopher emerge from the mansion and stroll across the grounds to visit Elvis' grave. The burial site is adorned with letters of grief, romantic poems, teddy bears and posthumous eulogies intended for the King, wherever he may be.

I don't read tabloids and I'm not big into conspiracy theories. I do believe Elvis is stone-cold dead. I don't expect to see him descending in a golden cloud of glory anytime soon, but as I reflect on the public offerings placed beside his tombstone, I can't help but think of how many people from all across the world still love this man. Too bad his friends couldn't save him from his addiction to prescription drugs. Hell, some of his friends enabled him to kill himself.

Unlike Elvis, I've had great support throughout my life, sometimes without me even realizing it. There were the family members who were there for me even when I was too sick or drugged up on pharmaceuticals to be there for them. Then there were the friends who risked lengthy jail sentences to provide me with medicine, before I received my medicine from the federal government. There were the nurses and doctors who took the time to listen, who fought for my access to cannabis and who saved my life. There were also journalists who cared enough to spend long hours with me and write articles that reflected the heart of my story and police officers who treated me with courtesy and respect, even when they did not fully comprehend the unique nature of my legal status. There were politicians who vocally supported and protected my constitutional rights. And of course, there were and still are scores of patients illegally obtaining their medicine, living in daily fear, who provide me with the reason to keep fighting. Finally, there were my fellow recipients of federal marijuana.

These people—some related to me by birth, some by friendship—came from all walks of life to sustain me through some of my darkest times. Even when they weren't physically present, I could envision them in my mind, which helped bring me out of deep depression when I was in so much pain and horribly ill.

They are all part of me, because they support my right to use medical cannabis and that's enough to qualify.

As I sit in the outdoor mall at Graceland, the faces of all the different people who have so positively affected my life and mission appear in my head like dusty pages in a scrapbook. Their voices echoing in the shadowy corners of my mind, I can still hear their stories in their own words...

IRVIN ROSENFELD - IND Patient #2

I'm a Florida stockbroker who handles multi-million dollar accounts while smoking twelve joints each day, supplied by the federal government. At the age of ten I was diagnosed with a disease that causes continuous growth of bone tumors. During my childhood and adolescence, I underwent seven operations to remove over thirty tumors. I had to be home-schooled through high school, because I couldn't even sit for more than ten minutes. The discomfort from the pressure on the growths was excruciating. As I grew into adulthood, I was always in constant pain from over 200 non-malignant tumors that press into the muscles at the ends of my long bones. I was initially treated with opiates, muscle relaxants and anti-inflammatory medications, which helped little and produced debilitating side effects. Finally, my physicians recommended cannabis.

My first experience with marijuana had been earlier in college. The first time I smoked a joint I didn't notice anything until I realized I'd been sitting without pain for half an hour, three times my normal limit. I knew then that there was something special about the drug, but I didn't realize that it had known medicinal value.

Later, when my doctors suggested cannabis, I did everything possible to use marijuana legally. I spoke with my local police chief to request access to confiscated marijuana to ease my symptoms. I designed a research protocol that was never funded, using myself as the lab rat. I testified to a Food and Drug Administration panel that marijuana enhanced the effects of opiates I was taking for pain control.

I was finally admitted to the federal program in 1982. Marijuana relaxes my tense muscles, allowing me to move with

much less pain. It also prevents the tumors from rupturing muscles and veins, which could cause me to bleed to death. As a legal
patient, I can affirm that when you have a devastating disease all
you care about is getting the right medicine and not having to
worry about being made a criminal. However, I have been treated
like a criminal by those who don't understand the laws that protect my right to use medicinal marijuana. One time, the treatment
I received was so atrocious, I was forced to a file a lawsuit. The
truth is almost impossible to believe.

I purchased a ticket for a flight from Fort Lauderdale to
Washington, D.C. I was traveling to our nation's capital to lend
my voice on behalf of patients and I planned to offer a "friend of
the court" brief before the United States Supreme Court. At the
time of the ticket purchase I informed airline representatives that
I would be flying with my federally prescribed medicine. I also
requested the airline's assistance in the event of an extended
flight delay. I need to smoke a joint about every two hours, so I
wanted to be sure that if my flight was grounded, I would be provided with an appropriate location to smoke my medicine in the
airport.

Prior to this occasion I had flown the same airline over a
dozen times and on every flight I was afforded reasonable accom-
modations. I was treated with dignity and respect on all previous
flights and so I expected no hassles.

On flight day, I arrived at the airport and checked in over
an hour early, informing the agent that I was disabled and would
need extra time to board my flight. The agent told me that it
wouldn't be a problem. Approximately thirty minutes before the
flight was scheduled to depart, I was paged and directed to speak
with the airline agents at the ticket counter, where I was summar-
ily informed that I wouldn't be permitted to fly to Washington with
my prescribed cannabis.

Upon hearing this, I showed them my prescription and the
brief that was to be argued the next day in the Supreme Court. I
explained that I had received my marijuana as part of a federal
government project that has existed for over twenty years. I told

the agent that I had never before been prohibited from flying with my medicine.

The agents informed me the decision to bar me was made by the airline's attorneys. The lawyers claimed to have only recently learned that I was carrying medical cannabis. They said that one of the reasons for the decision was that I didn't have express written permission to carry my medicine from the government of each state that the plane was to fly over. I tried to explain that the prescription, approved by the United States Drug Enforcement Administration, trumps any state requirement, but the airline employees would not listen to me.

After a lengthy discussion I was told that I wouldn't be permitted on the flight unless I left my medicine behind. I could not do that; I would have subjected myself to risk of injury if I needed my medicine during the trip and didn't have access to it. I asked to speak to the airline's attorneys, but was denied that request. Then I asked the airline agents to call the Broward County Sheriff's Office. The deputy who answered was familiar with my situation as I lived in Broward County, Florida, and explained to the airline agents that it was not illegal for me to carry federally-prescribed medicine on a plane no matter how many states it was to fly over. Regardless of the law enforcement official's explanation, the airline agents were adamant in their refusal to allow me to board the plane.

In the end, I was forced to book a last-minute flight on another airline at great expense and inconvenience to me. Clenching my teeth through the pain, I carried my heavy luggage all the way to another terminal without assistance. When I returned home from my trip, I sent a letter to the airline requesting that they issue an apology, reimburse me the additional money it cost to buy the ticket on the other airline and promise that such discrimination would never happen again. They refused. With my rights as a disabled traveler violated under the Air Carriers Access Act of 1986, I felt I had no recourse but to sue the airline.

Patients should not be forced to endure this type of treatment in "the land of the free." I am not a criminal. I am an American, albeit a sick American, who legally receives marijuana from the federal government. I deserve the same respect afforded any other citizen.

In spite of my struggles against discriminatory treatment like I suffered at the hands of the airline, I feel very fortunate. I appreciate what the government has done and hope it never stops. I'm vocal on this issue, because I want to educate people about why we should put this medicine in the hands of physicians, where it can do some good.

There are many people against us. Even as we educate the public, there are some people who are and always will be against us no matter what. People assume I'm always stoned out of my mind, smoking twelve joints a day for twenty-four years, but I have a responsible job handling millions of dollars. Thanks to marijuana, I am well enough to support myself, carry on the fight for my rights and try to help others who are too sick to help themselves or speak out. I hope our country will one day show more compassion for its gravely ill citizens.

ELVY MUSIKKA – IND Recipient #3

As a child I had congenital cataracts that required surgery. This produced a great deal of scar tissue, which eventually resulted in infected tear ducts. My ducts hold too many tears against the optic nerve at the back of my eye. This can and does cause permanent blindness if left untreated.

In 1975 I found out that I had glaucoma and by 1976 I was taking a number of prescribed medications. The side effects—tremendous headaches, pupil constriction to the point of blindness, lethargy, listlessness and depression—made my life as a single, working mother impossible to handle, so I stopped taking them. Finally, a doctor who was very compassionate told me that if I didn't start smoking marijuana soon, I would go blind.

I was thirty when I first smoked marijuana. I didn't even know how to inhale. It burned my throat so badly I thought I'd get throat cancer in no time. I was paranoid, because I had heard so many horrible stories about the dangers of marijuana.

I found another doctor who recommended that I eat the marijuana in brownies, since I was having trouble smoking. That worked well for four months and I was able to function normally. During that period, I was doing so well I even got a raise at work.

My doctor felt that with the kind of documentation we had, we could go to the research center at the University of Miami and persuade them to help me obtain legal marijuana. Instead, they offered a surgery that had only a 30 percent success rate.

I realize now that though I was not yet blinded by glaucoma, I and many others were blinded by ignorance. No one in their right mind would have gone through those surgeries if they knew that cannabis is one of the safest, most therapeutically active substances on this planet. Years ago, the American Medical Association originally objected to marijuana prohibition, because they knew it was a safe medicine for many people.

However, at the time, I didn't know any of this and I was concerned about the long-term effects of marijuana use, so I had the surgeries and spent the next twelve years living in hell. I lost so much of my sight that depression set in. I suffered from a lack of sleep, lack of appetite and I began drinking too much to numb the pain and sadness. It was a nightmare, a horror.

The only times I wasn't miserable were the few occasions when friends brought me marijuana. When they did, I felt better both physically and psychologically. I'd sleep at night and even have an appetite. A couple of times, I bought my own cannabis. It was considerably less expensive back then as opposed to today. I could purchase an ounce of really good stuff for about thirty dollars or cheaper varieties for twenty dollars, but even that was a strain on the budget of a single working mother trying to raise two children. Then I lost my job and my depression deepened. Once that happened, there just wasn't enough money for marijuana.

I became an experimental guinea pig for every conventional medicine being tested. One of the drugs actually worked for me for two years until I developed a resistance to it. I was soon left totally blind in my right eye.

In the early 1980s, after my children left home for college, I decided the only way I'd be able to get relief and not go broke was to grow my own marijuana. I began only growing the barest minimum, because I did not want to worry about the law. At the same time, I was still being treated conventionally. I went in for another unsuccessful surgery which finally resulted in total blindness.

Now I couldn't tell if it was day or night. Close your eyes. Can you still see the light through your eyelids? I couldn't. I ran into every piece of furniture and every wall in my house.

I continued growing and using marijuana and it kept my glaucoma under control. It eased my symptoms and even reversed some of my blindness. I could see again, but not well.

I knew it was time for me to find other people using medicinal marijuana. It was time for me to come out of hiding. Just as I was ready to start getting active, I was arrested for growing pot in March, 1988.

I had maybe three quarters of an ounce of dried herb, plus a plant that was starting to bud and two six-inch seedlings. That was it. For that, I faced five years in prison, $5000 in fines or both.

I had an overnight stay in jail that was most degrading. I immediately went public when I got out. I contacted every media outlet I could think of and I said, "Do you think this is right? I am going to be facing trial, because I don't want to go blind!"

I went to trial with the complete support of my community. There was no defense for medical marijuana in Florida and no laws to protect me. I was acquitted due to medical necessity. The judge sympathetically said that I would have to be insane not to do whatever I needed to save my sight. Leaving that courtroom, I felt that something wonderful had just happened.

While my trial was going on, with the assistance of Robert Randall, my doctors and attorneys applied to the federal government for me to have marijuana on an emergency basis. My doctor's request had twelve years of documentation to support it, yet the government totally ignored us.

Even after I was acquitted, the government still wouldn't give it to me, but I kept trying. I took to the airwaves and my attorney threatened to sue the federal government. I was finally accepted into the IND program and received my first marijuana cigarettes grown by the government on October 21, 1988.

When I became a legal smoker, there were only two individuals in the United States who were receiving medical marijuana through the federal government. One of them was Robert Randall, my hero of all time, because he was the first one to go through a trial and prove that he would be blind without it.

Being a legal smoker has more than its share of difficulties. Sometimes I need to smoke in a public place. I often have to hide what I'm doing. It seems ridiculous to me, but it's a small price to pay to have my health back.

In spite of all the struggles, I am a total optimist. I feel that the only enemy we really have is ignorance and I am confident that our ongoing fight to legalize medical marijuana will defeat that ignorance. As we bury the darkness of ignorance with the light of truth, there's going to be no opposition.

LARRY MONAGHAN – George's Friend

Being a broadcaster, I am accustomed to receiving strange calls in the middle of the night telling me to "Grab your camera and let's go!" So when George McMahon said he needed to go to Washington, D.C. to present a letter to the Department of Health and Human Services, I did not hesitate to accompany him.

I had my camera and two thermoses of coffee ready when George showed up. We packed up the truck and took off. Twenty-two hours later we unpacked the bags and checked into our rooms in a hotel in downtown Washington, D.C.

After a quick munch, a shower, and a few hours of sleep, the typical D.C. rush started. Fortunately we had a hot pot of coffee to start the day. Then it was on to the interviews and the announcement of a proposed schedule.

The first order of business was to make the press aware that George was in town to present a letter to then-director of Health and Human Services, Donna Shalala, as a protest for patients' rights.

George was not the only legal marijuana patient there that day. Irvin Rosenfeld attended as well, along with Frank Baker, a state worker from New Jersey who had been massively injured while working on a construction project. Frank had almost been ripped in half when he was caught in between pieces of a reinforcing rod. As an inspector for the state, it was his job to take such risks. After years of surgeries, drugs and being confined to a wheelchair, a "friend" had asked the injured man if he'd ever heard of medical marijuana. One thing led to another and Frank obtained a small amount. The marijuana stimulated his appetite, not only for food but for life itself.

Until his introduction to medical marijuana, Frank, a life-long Republican and staunch supporter of the war on drugs, had been contemplating any method necessary to end his own existence. Within months of starting treatment with medical marijuana, he was able to get out of his wheelchair for the first time in years. His doctors were amazed and tried to get Frank into the federal IND program. His request was denied, because the government had closed the program and was accepting no new admissions. As far as they were concerned, the government knew all they needed to know about the "killer weed" and no more new studies would be done. They did offer him a substitute in Marinol, but this quickly put him back in a wheelchair.

All three patients, our camera crew, CNN, three television channels, the crew from Patients Out of Time and members of other organizations who care about the treatment of sick people, were there to let people know that the federal program had been shut down. The decision to close the program was economic as well as political, because the only legal producer of cannabis was a small farm in Mississippi and the government couldn't supply the drug to more than a few patients.

George, Irvin and Frank arrived at the front door of the Department of Health and Human Services. They were politely asked to leave, but were allowed to hand over their letter of demands for patients' rights. The guard at the door summoned the local police, who asked everyone to please leave "government property." Everyone moved to the street corner, where George and the other patients gave interviews to the media before we packed up the truck and headed home.

The doctors had told George he wasn't going to live, but twelve years after being admitted to the government program, he is still asking why other people with similar needs are dying painful, expensive deaths because of a policy that declares cannabis use to be a sin.

DARRELL PAULSEN – George's Friend

I live with cerebral palsy, diagnosed about eight months after my birth and I suffer from intense muscle spasms. I have little or no use of my legs and my left arm might as well be nonexistent, since I am unable to do much of anything with it. I live my life from a parlor wheelchair. I first realized that cannabis was helping my symptoms at the age of seventeen, when I used it to treat my chronic constipation. Now I use marijuana primarily to treat my spasms. It has always been effective medicine for me.

Over the past twelve years, I have known George McMahon as both a patient and a person. Even though George and I both use medical marijuana to treat our symptoms, I think we would have become good friends regardless of our status as patients.

I met George in 1990, when I was only nineteen. We were both living in Iowa at the time and we were attending a medical marijuana conference, sponsored by NORML and the Grass Roots Party. Before I met George, I was aware of the Compassionate IND Program, but I did not know the specific details about how it was implemented. By the time I found a doctor who was sympathetic and supportive, the program had already been shut down by the Bush administration, so I never had the opportunity to apply. I certainly could have met the requirements of the protocol if it was still open.

I was overwhelmed when I first got to know George. Here was a man who had recently evaded death. He had only been receiving his government marijuana for a short time, yet his spirits were high. It was empowering to meet such a person.

George has been a true friend to me. He has the qualities of a leader and he is somebody I look up to. If it had not been for him, I would not have done the things I have done for as long as I have done them.

George was the man who finally convinced me to cut my hair and wear a suit, but I have since forgiven him for this. In fact, it was probably one of the best things I did in my entire life. The new look made me more approachable and respectable to politicians and other officials. In fact, it allowed me to have a lot of great experiences that I might not have had otherwise. For example, I go up to the Minnesota State Capitol three or four times each week as an advocate for people with disabilities. Now when I roll into a legislator's office, clean cut and respectful, I can meet the congressman as a fellow citizen.

George's legal status is inspiring to me. Sometimes it can be kind of intimidating, because he is legally allowed to do what I do illegally, without having to worry about all the repercussions.

I have finally reached the point where I believe that wherever I happen to be in my life, I am home. I will take my medicine wherever and whenever I need to, even in the middle of a crowded street if necessary.

My main goal is to be an activist to empower people, especially those who are young. We have so much power if we can just find the courage to use it. We have the right to vote and the freedom to get involved in our local communities. We have a responsibility to know our representatives, those movers and shakers who can get things done. Once we develop relationships with them, we can continually build on those friendships to help provide the services and programs that sick, disabled and senior citizens need to survive and have rich and fulfilling lives.

With the current level of public support and legislation, I think more patients are speaking out. It still takes a lot of courage to risk their healthcare, housing, education and transportation. These are all things that people who aren't disabled take for granted on a daily basis, but medical marijuana patients are forced to consider it. I feel pretty confident that I have helped patients to feel more comfortable talking to their doctors or healthcare providers, whether they use marijuana occasionally or on a regular basis.

Over the last couple of years, I think the law enforcement community is beginning to understand that marijuana has medical benefits, but they are still entangled with regulations. Whether those regulations are enforced is dependent on the political leanings of the local administration.

In my home state of Minnesota, the law enforcement community, the commissioner of public safety and the commissioner of health are behind me. They all want to support those who need medical marijuana, but political consequences are a major concern. Minnesota state lawmakers have actually expressed the desire to gain the authority to implement medical marijuana programs, assuming that they can find funding, researchers and permission from the federal government.

I live with disability. I deal with it every day. I know that I am different from most other people and I have slowly learned to accept and even celebrate this part of me.

JOHN MARKES – George's Friend

I am a thirty-nine year old veteran. I've been disabled since 1986 and homebound for the last few years. My current medical problems prevent me from working and I am forced to spend most of my time resting or recuperating from the minimal exertions my disabilities will allow. Buying groceries, washing a glass, getting into bed or even bathing are agonies I endure on an everyday basis.

While serving in the military, I was trained as an electronics technician and a nuclear reactor operator. I was medically discharged from the Navy in 1987. I later enrolled in a local university, but was forced to withdraw in late 1994 as my health rapidly declined due to excessive weight loss. I had started out at a healthy 200 pounds in August 1993; by the time I withdrew in September and despite the efforts of my physicians, my weight plummeted to a mere 146 pounds. During this period, I had been receiving my care at a VA Hospital. In August of 1993, the hospital's gastroenterology department began to treat me for severe diarrhea. A short time later, other symptoms arose which included anorexia, nausea and unbearable stomach pains. Some of the pain was alleviated when the doctors discovered and got rid of a series of internal infections. Yet I still had no appetite and the severe nausea and diarrhea continued.

After losing even more weight, one of my doctors informed me that they had exhausted their options in conventional drugs and therapies. My doctor discreetly told me that marijuana might be an avenue to consider for better treatment. I went to the hospital's medical library and looked up medical marijuana to learn more about it.

I was amazed to discover a huge amount of positive information about this stereotypically "bad" drug. In fact, it was the only thing listed in the Merck Manual (at that time) for weight gain. Two months later, I had lost an additional twenty pounds and was faced with a life-or-death decision: try the only medication that might help or rely on the failing treatments the doctors were providing. After much prayer and thought, I procured some marijuana and smoked it. After a couple smoking sessions, I noticed my pain and nausea disappear and I developed a classic case of the "munchies"—a truly unusual experience for someone who typically has no appetite at all. I began to see such an improvement that I stopped using my other medications.

A few weeks later when I went to see my doctors, they were amazed at my recovery. I told them about my marijuana use. They told me to continue with my new method of medication. At last I was able to exercise again and eat a healthy diet. However, in 1997, I had my home searched by the police. The authorities questioned me and I explained the medicinal benefits the marijuana they found provided for me. I was put under arrest and a court case ensued. In response to these legal problems, my primary care provider at the VA hospital reviewed my case jointly with a local university medical center. They concluded that marijuana was my only option.

Since then, I've continued to use marijuana, though I'm forced to buy it on the black market. The main problem I face is the cost. I spend one-fifth of my income on the drug. Currently, I am petitioning the VA hospital to provide me with medical marijuana. My status is stalled in a conflict between my doctors and the State of Arkansas. My doctors say "Use it" and the state says "Don't you dare!"

I was a lifelong bodybuilding enthusiast, but because of the extensive damage to my joints, I am not able to work out as much as I would like. Nevertheless, working out is a prescribed part of my medical treatment. My doctors want me to gain as much weight as I can, so that in the event of rapid weight loss, I have a reserve to work with. It is difficult, however, because I can't accomplish this therapy on my own. I need assistance with lifting any kind of weight and often I don't have anyone to help me. It can be very frustrating.

When I'm not at the VA hospital, I am usually confined to the rooms of my apartment. My apartment is not adapted for disabled people, but I still feel lucky to have secured this residence. Many places in town would not rent to me, because I have a prior conviction for marijuana possession. I'm lucky to have a bird and three cats to keep my company during the long stretches when I'm alone in my apartment.

I am always discreet about using my medicine, but this is difficult to accomplish sometimes. After all, I can't exactly blow smoke out my apartment window or let people outside see me take my medicine. I always ensure that the windows and blinds are closed and everything is locked. This helps to protect me, but it makes me feel even more isolated from the world than I already am.

Another challenge I face is vulnerability. I worry about being a target of people from both sides of the law, dealers and police officers. An officer might arrest me and a dealer might rob me. Sometimes I feel like a sitting duck. In fact, one dealer recently took three hundred dollars from me, promising to provide me with medicine, but never did. This person left me in a terrible situation: empty-handed and facing many days filled with pain, loss of functioning and weight loss. Living on my veteran's benefits, I simply can't afford to purchase more medicine if a dealer rips me off.

The funny thing is, I use marijuana to feel normal and healthy, whereas those using it recreationally are just trying to get high. That's the medicine in marijuana. It alleviates all the symptoms of my digestive disorder, even stimulating a normal appetite. So when someone argues that people who use medical marijuana "just want to get high" I tell them, "No, they just want to feel normal."

JUNE – George's Mother

George was a lovable little baby and he was very easy to take care of. I really never had too much trouble with him. I was a single mother, working all the time, but my other children assisted me with raising him. I also had babysitters from time to time. When he was very young, I hired a German woman to help take care of him. He learned to speak German before he learned English.

At the time of George's birth, I already knew that I had an unusual bone structure in my hands and I noticed that George shared this trait. I never thought anything about it. I thought it was just an unusual characteristic, like a birthmark. Then I discovered that, like his older brother, George could not straighten out his arm. I consented to let a doctor perform surgery on his arm, but it didn't help. I never thought about the possibility of a genetic condition and I had never heard of Nail Patella Syndrome.

As a toddler, my little George was sick much of the time. One time he had rheumatic fever and I was so scared that he might not live through it. He was in the hospital many times and whenever I brought him home my mother came to help me nurse him back to health. He was often bedridden for months at a time.

His illnesses were difficult for me, because I worked by appointments. I was constantly rearranging my schedule around his needs. He had a phone right by his bed so he could call me if he needed me. I didn't mind; I would have done anything for my George, but a few of my clients were not so understanding.

George was always a very good child during these periods of illness. He enjoyed reading and watching television and he liked to color with crayons. He preferred for things to be quiet while he was sick.

George was so glad when he could finally go back to school after a long bout of sickness. One year, he asked if he could take a wrestling class. I was hesitant to let him participate in such strenuous physical activity, but I didn't want to stifle him so I let him give it a try. Day after day, he came home dragging and weary after his wrestling class. I soon put a stop to it, telling him that he was not to get involved in high-impact sports anymore, because it was too hard on his heart.

Later, George got interested in ice-skating and roller-skating. The cardiovascular aspect wasn't as hard on him as wrestling, so I encouraged him to continue. When he wasn't doing that, he was an avid reader. His reading certainly paid off. In the seventh grade, George won the spelling contest in his school. His teacher encouraged him to enter a state competition, but he wouldn't do it, because he was shy and didn't want to be in the spotlight.

Even though he was not as healthy as his siblings, I still required George to do little chores around the house when he was a kid. He took out the trash, folded towels, raked the yard and mowed the lawn. These jobs didn't hurt him any and that helped him to feel good about himself.

I did not know about George's cannabis use until he was already accepted into the federal program. I didn't like the fact that he was using it at first. To me, it seemed like he was just abusing drugs. It took me a while to understand his condition and why he needed marijuana. When I saw how he was getting healthier, I had to admit that marijuana is medicine. By using it under a doctor's orders and supervision, I think he is doing the right thing. I would be concerned if he was going out in the streets for his medicine.

Both of George's older bothers are very judgmental about his medicine. I tell them, "You aren't around him. You don't know." I understand their concerns and hesitation though. I raised them and I'm very much against drug abuse. I get so mad just thinking about how it devastates people's lives.

However, after seeing what marijuana has done for my son, I firmly believe it should be made available for medical use. I am all for people getting what they need to be healthy and well. If a person uses marijuana for medical reasons, then I support it. Studies are showing that there is so much medicine in the marijuana leaf. Scientists just need to discover how they can use it. I think all states should have a program for patients. Nevertheless, I feel it should be strictly regulated.

I don't mind my son smoking marijuana anymore. He doesn't smoke his medicine here in my home, out of respect for me. We go out on the front porch when he needs to smoke his medicine.

I am proud of my son. I never had any trouble with him lying. He was always honest with everything he said. He has had a hard time in life because of his sickness, but he has raised three great kids.

George has always wanted to accomplish more. He had something to prove. He has done and learned a lot of different things. No matter what he did, he learned. In spite of what he learned, it never stopped him from taking risks. When you think about it, that's how he got his medicine.

JENNIFER – George's Daughter

I was seventeen when my dad first was admitted to the medical marijuana program. His illness was something we kids thought about every morning when we woke up. It was pretty hard on all of us. It was on our minds all the time. We missed out on a lot because of it. There were many activities in which my dad could not participate.

During 1989, when he came home from the hospital, we saw firsthand the different effects the smoking had on him versus the prescription drugs. Sometimes he was practically in a coma with all the regular medication and pills. He didn't even know who we were. He was completely out of it.

Whenever he smoked, on the other hand, he could participate in life and he wasn't as stressed or in pain. It brought him out of that comatose state. He was happier and it positively affected the whole family. We started getting along with each other better, because we were not as stressed.

I helped administer treatments for my dad, like cleaning out his infections. I accepted it at the time, because it was just something I had to do. When I got older, I resented it more. There were times when I thought I shouldn't have that intense responsibility at such a young age.

I definitely grew up more quickly than most kids. My siblings and I became very responsible adults because of my dad's illness and his use of medical marijuana. Most people accept his use of pot and are fine with it. The people who don't agree with it won't ask questions about in the first place to learn more; they've already made up their minds. The people who ask questions are willing to learn, willing to see a different point of view and actually are concerned about us as people.

I didn't talk about my dad's medicine before he was legal. Once he became legal, it was easier to talk to people about his condition and treatment. I have seen enough to know that it is very helpful, but I also know that lots of people just smoke it to get high. That makes me mad because those irresponsible people hinder patients from getting the quality medicine they need.

In a way, it surprised me that the government would provide marijuana for my dad. I knew it was medicine, but medical use of marijuana was not talked about at that time. It's definitely improved my dad's health and the quality of life for him and my entire family.

LINDA – George's Daughter

From 1985 until about 1990, my dad was really sick, even to the point of being at death's door. His joints were swollen with inflammation. He stayed in bed for days at a time.

I have Nail Patella Syndrome, too, so I never participated in sports when I was a child. I get severe muscle spasms and swollen joints and I have glaucoma. All of these symptoms have been linked to the Nail Patella gene.

My youngest daughter also has Nail Patella Syndrome, but we aren't sure yet how this might affect her later in life. We know she has kidney problems, since one kidney is larger than the other. We don't know if that will cause significant problems for her down the road. Only time will tell. From what we can observe at this point, she is just a little underweight, but otherwise is developing normally.

When I was growing up, I just took aspirin and other over-the-counter painkillers to manage my pain. Now that I'm older and the pain is more intense, I take powerful prescription painkillers when my knees and joints are inflamed and muscle relaxers for my spasms.

It was really tough growing up with a sick father. When my dad took the heavy-duty painkillers, it seemed like he slept all the time. It made him really grumpy and he threw up a lot. I think it frustrated him that he could not function normally. He wanted to be involved with my siblings and me, but the illness was just too much for him. I never held it against him, because I could see how sick he was. Our whole family knew he was in constant, debilitating pain.

When I was in high school I had to deal with friends who did not understand why my father smoked marijuana. They used to tease me about my dad. They called him a pothead, even when he was smoking legally. They thought he smoked in order to get high, but I've never known my dad to smoke for that reason. He always smoked just to feel better. It took a couple of years before they could accept that for my father, marijuana was medicine.

It is so much different now. Fifteen years ago the media hardly ever talked about medical marijuana, but now the issue is in the papers regularly. This has made it easier on me, because now people are more quick to grasp the idea that my dad uses cannabis for medical reasons, not recreational. When I first tell people that my dad smokes medical marijuana, they usually ask me if he has cancer, because that is what they have heard reporters cover in their stories.

I've never used marijuana, so I don't know if it would work for me, but I certainly wish that I had the legal right to try it. The prescription painkillers I have knock me out, so I stay away from them except in the most severe cases. I can't be a functional mother to my little girl if I'm sleeping all the time.

I know some people might disagree with using marijuana, but I have seen its positive benefits firsthand. I have seen what it has done for my dad. I am grateful that marijuana was made legally available to my father. He would have been dead without it.

ORLISS – George's Friend; a Librarian and Church Organist
I've known George for over ten years. He's one of the most honest people I know. I would trust him with anything. He's just one of those rare individuals to whom kindness comes naturally.

Before I met George, I never knew anybody who used and benefited from medical cannabis. Although I was somewhat ignorant of the facts, I have an open mind so I had no problem with his use of medical marijuana.

I lived in the same town as George for many years. He often came into the public library where I work. He was virtually a permanent fixture there. He used our Internet service a lot to do research in his efforts to promote the issue of medical marijuana. I've heard George speak on the issue in public several times and I was very impressed.

Even though we lived in a tiny town in Iowa, I never heard much gossip about him. I think people were really quite accepting of his condition and treatment.

Before George got his marijuana from the federal government, I never heard of cannabis being used medically. It just wasn't a topic that came up in discussion. The issue frequently catches my attention now.

My opinion about marijuana changed after knowing George, because I now think there are many cases in which it is truly a medical necessity.

I don't understand why the government has a problem with cannabis. It's not a chemical that has been altered by man. It's just a plant. Sure, some people abuse it. However, just as many or more misuse prescription drugs. It's easier to acquire prescription substances and it's more socially acceptable to take them. The hemp plant, on the other hand, is natural.

When George first started coming into the library, he was not in good health. There were long stretches when I would not see him at all. I'd hear from others that he was laid up at home and unable to get up or leave his house. I think he is stronger now. I remember there were times when he absolutely could not walk without a cane. Now he uses a cane only occasionally, if at all. I think his health has been relatively stable over the last four years.

I once talked with some people in our town who suspected George was dealing or selling pot. I told them the federal government program is so strict that George would not do anything to jeopardize his place in the program. He is very responsible with his medicine.

Medical marijuana is a touchy subject for some people, but I don't really understand why. Look around at some of the things going on in the world. I think that the government is being petty with their concerns about patients being criminals.

"George! George! Snap out of it!" Margaret's voice finally breaks my reverie and returns my brain to planet earth.

"Sorry, I was just thinking about.... Never mind that, how was Graceland? All you dreamed and more?"

Margaret beams. "It was amazing. I wish you could have seen the grave up close and the inside of the mansion."

"Yeah, it was pretty cool, George." Christopher tries to act nonchalant, but I can see through his charade. He's practically bubbling with the enthusiasm of a little boy who has just gotten off Space Mountain at Disney World.

The two of them chatter on, describing each room in detail from floor to ceiling. I smile, not so much at the images of Graceland's interior that their words evoke, but at the beauty of two people—two among many—who have improved my life by their presence and support. I smile because I am a lucky man.

A Long Strange Trip...
Where Do We Go From Here?

The future depends on what we do in the present.

– Mohandas Gandhi

One of the most conservative, state-funded colleges in America is growing marijuana. There is hope yet.

We arrived in Mississippi this afternoon. I stand outside the twelve foot-high barbed wire fence encasing Uncle Sam's marijuana garden. We're almost at the end of the green path. Who would have thought that the federal government would be contracting state employees as pot growing experts? Over the past thirty-four years, thousands of pounds of *cannabis sativa* have passed through the security gates. Some of it goes to provide the IND patients with medical marijuana and some of it is used to train drug-sniffing police dogs to aid in the arrest of drug dealers, buyers and users, as well as medical marijuana patients unlucky enough to have been barred from the IND program. The same government project that saved my life is also used to destroy the lives of other patients. It's a lethal irony, that's for sure.

The National Institute of Drug Abuse has denied me permission to enter the garden, even though no marijuana is growing inside the gates on this particular day. Politicians, scientists, educators and doctors are all given regular access to a field full of government cannabis. The administrative researchers even hire local college students to enter the compound, in order to harvest the mature cannabis crop, providing they submit to a search upon leaving the farm. No reporters are allowed inside the barbed wire, however, and no patients. I can smoke the marijuana grown at this garden, but I can't see the field of dirt it's grown in.

It's hard to hope at times. Somewhere a patient is in chains, a brilliant mind is bound by shackles of ignorance, a candle flickers and burns out. Sometimes I don't know which is louder, the screams of the dying or the silence of the dead.

I'm not sure what the answer is, but there's one thing I know for certain. The solution does not lie in treating everyone the same or in forcing all people to assimilate and adhere to one rigid definition of "what is right." As e.e. cummings wrote, "To be nobody but yourself, in a world which is doing its best, night and day, to make you everybody else, means to fight the hardest battle which any human being can fight; and never stop fighting."

On February 12, 2002, President Bush declared an intensification of the anti-drug crusade, claiming that his administration would reduce illegal drug use by 25 percent. The next day, federal narcotics agents dynamited the front door of a state-mandated medical marijuana clinic that served more than two hundred patients each day, the Sixth Street Harm Reduction Center in San Francisco. They seized over six hundred plants and made several arrests, including that of writer and publisher Ed Rosenthal and Richard Watts, the executive director of the clinic. These men were charged with cultivating more than one hundred plants and maintaining a place to grow marijuana. If convicted, these men could face forty years in prison.

San Francisco police officials refused to participate in the raids and made public statements to that effect. District Attorney Terence Hallinan stood on the steps of the Commonwealth Club and said, "Matters of health and safety are for the local government and not some federal, national agency. It's a decision to be made by the voters of California. I call on the DEA to respect the wishes of the people of California and stay out of the marijuana clubs of San Francisco."

City Supervisor Mark Leno stated, "These raids are a

direct assault on the health care system of the city and county of San Francisco. The DEA's outrageous action today is also a direct assault on the citizens of California who in 1996, by a near 70 percent majority, voted in support of the compassionate use of medical cannabis. There is absolutely no reason why the federal government should be prohibiting law abiding citizens from accessing the medicine they need for their health and well-being."

The angry response by members of the public showed they concurred. One man stood with his arms crossed and repeatedly tore up the yellow tape surrounding the "crime scene," much to the irritation of the DEA officers.

Twelve hours after the raid, DEA Chief Asa Hutchinson gave a speech titled, "Let's Not Punt on the Third Down," a football analogy referring to the drug war. Initially the police had threatened to eject any hecklers in the crowd; they didn't expect that almost the entire crowd would be comprised of angry patients and their supporters. When Hutchison claimed that science had shown no medical benefit to marijuana, patients looked right in his face and called him a liar.

The speech moderator said that he was going to choose a balanced set of questions and comments from the audience, but after reviewing the stack of about 300 question cards, he informed the crowd that there appeared to be no support for the DEA. He said he would have to let Hutchinson's speech represent the DEA side of the issue and stick to questions with an anti-DEA perspective.

The audience brought up some provocative questions. One person said, "I am a Vietnam veteran and my doctor recommends I smoke pot to ease the symptoms of my ongoing, debilitating medical condition. I get great relief from using it. Can you tell me what I'm supposed to do now?"

Another person asked, "Given the 400,000 to zero yearly fatality ratio, plus the established benefits of THC, why isn't tobacco a Schedule I drug?" Asa Hutchinson responded that Congress has seen fit to establish certain drugs as legal, others as illegal, within certain "parameters of social mores."

DEA spokesman Richard Meyer claimed, "We've said all

along the cultivation and distribution of marijuana is illegal regardless of state or local law." He obviously didn't know about the federal government's marijuana garden. Or he didn't want anyone else to know about it.

Some government officials have a lot to learn. As long as they're willing to listen, I want to make the truth known.

It's really scary for so many sick people who need marijuana but fear going to jail. In "Legal Issues Related to the Medical Use of Marijuana," Kevin Zeese succinctly explains the dilemma. "Seriously ill Americans are faced with a difficult choice if they need cannabis as medicine—they can either obey the law and suffer the consequences of their illness and perhaps die or they can break the law and face criminal prosecution. Similarly, healthcare professionals caring for patients who could benefit from cannabis also face a difficult choice. They can either hide information from their patients on the medical benefits of cannabis or they can tell their patients about its medical utility and advise them to break the law."

Patients in need and physicians who understand the value of medical marijuana both are caught between a rock and a hard place. I know that marijuana is not a panacea. But it has been used medically for thousands of years. Each patient has a unique physiology and not every person benefits from it nor should every person use marijuana. It is not known to actually cure any specific disease or disorder. It does, however, in many patients, control certain symptoms such as nausea, pain, stress and spasms. Some people can become emotionally dependent, but this emotional dependency revolves around the person's use of the herb, not the cannabis itself.

The issue becomes more complicated when considering the multiple and often conflicting uses of drugs. Most drugs can be used in ways that heal and ways that harm. Alcohol can intoxicate and destroy a liver, but it can also cleanse a wound and some reports say it benefits the heart. Tobacco may cause lung cancer, but it can also extract the venom from a bee sting. Opiates can cause extreme addiction but also relieve acute pain. Cocaine can induce a heart attack, but it can also provide an effective topical stimulant during cardiac surgery. Problems do not arise because of the substances themselves, but because of the manner in which they are used. Some people may use marijuana as an excuse for their negative choices, but cannabis can literally save a person's life—like it saved mine.

Over the course of the many years I've worked to educate people about medical marijuana, I've received thousands of letters. They come from all over the world, including Yugoslavia, Thailand, England, Canada and Holland. The people who write these letters come from every walk of life. They are legislators, doctors, lawyers, professors, good Samaritans and even children. Some are college students wanting help on medical marijuana term papers. Out of all these letters, I feel the most important words are those penned by the patients themselves.

I have received sincere expressions of thanks from patients who legally participate in state marijuana programs, but fear federal prosecution. People have kept me in their prayers, calling me everything from "the nicest man" to an "angel of hope" in their letters. One woman suffering from a neuromuscular disorder wrote, "People like you give me the courage to fight and hold my head up high in spite of my disability. Thank you so much for simply being who you are. You are an inspiration to many people."

I try to be grateful, though I don't accept their assessments. I'm just a man. If life had not dealt me such a bizarre hand, I probably wouldn't be concerned with the issue of medical marijuana.

People have written to me seeking information on medical marijuana treatment for rheumatoid arthritis and fibromyalgia, cancer, paraplegia, quadriplegia, AIDS, endometriosis, post-traumatic stress disorder and chronic pelvic and back pain. One spinal cord injury patient stated, "I can't believe the government of this country can't see the difference between heroin and a kind, gentle, caressing medicine that not only heals the body but the soul as well."

Patients running out of time often write to share their daily struggles. I do my best to empathize, although being a legal smoker puts me in a much better situation than many patients out there on their own. Consider the story of one sick woman who recently contacted me. She started smoking marijuana about six years ago for pain, but she no longer can afford it. She lives in Washington state where it can be prescribed legally, however, she can't find a doctor that will even talk to her about it because of fears of prosecution under federal law.

Then there's another young woman who wrote to tell me about her struggles with multiple scleroris. She used cannabis in the past for relief, but like so many others, her company has instituted a drug testing policy.

Still another woman who has fibromyalgia wrote in a state of panic and desperation. When she told her doctors about her marijuana use to relieve her pain, they indicated on her medical records that she had an addiction problem. Now, her doctors won't prescribe her any pain medication because of her status and so she endures intense physical pain with no medication of any kind. This has left her unable to work and she fears she will be evicted from her home soon.

Reading these stories of desperation written by people who've lost hope and have nowhere to turn is difficult to do. They are suffering while I'm lucky to be in the IND program. Most patients are simply trying to make it through another day. I don't have to fight to live and I don't really even like to fight people who might turn out to be my friends. I have already won my battle with the bureaucrats. The government grows, packages and ships my marijuana prescription. I could sit back and be quiet if I wanted to.

Many federal officials would prefer that I do just that: sit back and be quiet. They don't want people making waves. But I have sworn that so long as there is breath in my body, so long as patients are being jailed and destroyed and so long as people are willing to listen, I will continue to tell my story. At times, when I feel defeated or worn out, I just think about all the patients who need me to speak for them. I think about the ongoing battle, the ups and downs, the wins and losses. I think of what Margaret Thatcher once said: "You may have to fight a battle more than once to win it." And then I carry on.

I recently received a wonderful letter from a Canadian friend and patient. My heart soared as my eyes moved over the page.

My Dear George:

I wanted you to be the first to know that today I received, via special delivery courier, my acceptance under the Exemption 56 Health Canada Program.

Believe me George, as I write to you, tears are flooding my eyes. I am so damned happy! I know I have told you before, but it bears repeating. Via some twist of fate, I found out I had Nail Patella Syndrome in December of 1999, and I was in terrible pain, virtually useless and bedridden for two years. Then I found the NPS sites, which led me to the educational website that contained your story and the hope you offered. Your kind and generous sharing of your experiences and knowledge with me, for my doctor's information, made this happen, George.

I am so much better since using the plant, more active, happier, calmer, and more flexible, and I am actually enjoying my life! What were the odds of finding you, George? "Thank you" doesn't say it enough. Be sure in knowing that what you have been able to achieve through your persistence has also benefitted this Canadian girl and the world!

Love to you and yours,
Linda Moseby, Exemptee.

Reading her words left me breathless. She has expressed what the medical marijuana movement is ultimately about: one person demonstrates compassion towards another, dispelling ignorance with enlightened knowledge.

Afterwards, I realized things had come full circle. All the pain I endured throughout the early years of my life was suddenly imbued with a new sense of dignity and meaning. If my experiences blazed a trail for others, then the journey was worth every moment, even the agonizing ones.

Years of intense struggle have granted me personal knowledge of the harsh realities of life. Yet I retain a strangely resilient sense of hope and idealism. I feel like a tiny pebble tossed into still waters, rippling outwards.

Taoists say that water is the most solid substance on earth. When rushing against a rock, water softly yields, but over time that liquid will erode even the hardest of stones. People often change in much the same manner. I've always preferred the soft touch, myself. It's much more effective than blatant, "in-your-face" activism.

Compassion, like cruelty, can have a human face. If we reach out to one person at a time, and that person in turn spreads the message to others, then we will succeed in making tomorrow better than today and the suffering of persecuted patients will not have been in vain.

As Christopher, Margaret and I stroll away from Uncle Sam's marijuana garden, I am left with the nagging sense that our journey is not complete. Not that I expected closure. I've learned much from the past, but I'm more concerned with the future. Where will the green path take us? I don't have an exact answer, but I think the path will lead us to a good place if we are humble and strong enough to follow it.

Green is the color of life. It carries the promise of renewal and rebirth. It reminds me of cannabis flowers, emeralds, iguanas and river moss.

I'm no rolling stone. When I get home, I'm going to take it easy in order to regain my strength. Silence and solitude are what I need. Time to recuperate and process things. No interviews, legislators, activists, students, cops or cameras for a while. I'll kiss Margaret, pet the dog, plant some flowers and light a government joint. I'll throw out a net or a hook into the river and see what I can catch.

But I'll be returning to the fray soon to fight for those suffering who cannot speak for themselves and whose pain may be alleviated like mine—by medical cannabis. Then I'll be fishing for hearts and minds.

Epilogue

Since returning from the journey that took us from Little Rock to Memphis to Uncle Sam's marijuana field in Mississippi, the delta-9-tetrahydrocannabinol (THC) content of my government cannabis has been decreased from .4% to .3% or less on average. Thus, my dose has been cut by 25 percent or more. No government officials ever contacted my doctor ahead of time to inform him of the change. My doctor's last shipment contained a form with the lower percentage count, along with a brief explanation stating the reason: street marijuana only averages .3% THC, so a patient doesn't need more. According to the government, nobody "needs" street marijuana, so I'm a little baffled as to why they are using it as a benchmark for a suitable amount of medical marijuana that I and so many others need to alleviate pain and suffering. In any case, since smoking this last batch I've suffered from nausea, night sweats, pain, sleeplessness and decreased mobility.

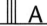
Appendix

Chronic Cannabis Use in the Compassionate Investigational New Drug Program: An Examination of Benefits and Adverse Effects of Legal Clinical Cannabis

Ethan Russo, Mary Lynn Mathre, Al Byrne, Robert Velin, Paul J. Bach, Juan Sanchez-Ramos and Kristin A. Kirlin

Journal of Cannabis Therapeutics, Vol. 2 (1)

Ethan Russo, Robert Velin, and Paul J. Bach are affiliated with Montana Neuro-behavioral Specialists, 900 North Orange Street, Missoula, MT 59802 USA

Mary Lynn Mathre and Al Byrne are affiliated with Patients Out of Time, 1472 Fish Pond Road, Howardsville, VA 24562 USA (E-mail: Patients@medicalcannabis.com).

Juan Sanchez-Ramos is affiliated with the Department of Neurology, University of South Florida, Tampa, USA.

Kristin A. Kirlin is affiliated with the Department of Psychology, University of Montana, Missoula, MT 59812.

ABSTRACT. The Missoula Chronic Clinical Cannabis Use Study was proposed to investigate the therapeutic benefits and adverse effects of prolonged use of "medical marijuana" in a cohort of seriously ill patients.

Use of cannabis was approved through the Compassionate Investigational New Drug (IND) program of the Food and Drug Administration (FDA). Cannabis is obtained from the National Institute on Drug Abuse (NIDA), and is utilized under the supervision of a study physician.

The aim of this study is to examine the overall health status of 4 of the 7 surviving patients in the program. This project provides the first opportunity to scrutinize the long-term effects of cannabis on patients who have used a known dosage of a standardized, heat-sterilized quality-controlled supply of low-grade marijuana for 11 to 27 years.

Results demonstrate clinical effectiveness in these patients in treating glaucoma, chronic musculoskeletal pain, spasm and nausea, and spasticity of multiple sclerosis. All 4 patients are stable with respect to their chronic conditions, and are taking many fewer standard pharmaceuticals than previously.

Mild changes in pulmonary function were observed in 2 patients, while no functionally significant attributable sequelae were noted in any other physiological system examined in the study, which included: MRI scans of the brain, pulmonary function tests, chest X-ray, neuropsychological tests, hormone and immunological assays, electroencephalography, P300 testing, history, and neurological clinical examination.

These results would support the provision of clinical cannabis to a greater number of patients in need. We believe that cannabis can be a safe and effective medicine with various suggested improvements in the existing Compassionate IND program.

INTRODUCTION
The Missoula Chronic Clinical Cannabis Use Study was proposed to investigate the therapeutic benefits and adverse effects of prolonged use of "medical marijuana" in a cohort of seriously ill patients approved through the Compassionate Investigational New Drug (IND) program of the Food and Drug Administration (FDA) for legal use of cannabis obtained from the National Institute on Drug Abuse (NIDA), under the supervision of a study physician. The aim was to examine the overall health status of 8 surviving patients in the program. Four patients were able to take part, while three wished to remain anonymous, and one was too ill to participate. Unfortunately, that person, Robert Randall, succumbed to his condition during the course of the study. Thus, 7 surviving patients in the USA remain in the Compassionate IND program.

Despite the obvious opportunity to generate data on the use of cannabis and its possible sequelae in these patients, neither NIDA, other branches of the National Institutes of Health, nor the FDA has published an analysis of information from this cohort. An examination of the contents of the National Library of Medicine Database (PubMed), and search engines of NIDA employing multiple combinations of key words failed to retrieve a single citation. The Missoula Chronic Cannabis Use Study thus provides a unique and important opportunity to scrutinize the long-term effects of cannabis on patients who have used a known dosage of standardized, heat-sterilized quality-controlled supply of low-grade medical marijuana for 11 to 27 years. The results are compared to those of past chronic use studies in an effort to gain insight into the benefits and sequelae of this controversial agent in modern health care.

PREVIOUS CHRONIC CANNABIS USE STUDIES

The first systematic modern study of chronic cannabis usage was the *Indian Hemp Drugs Commission Report* at the end of the 19th century (Kaplan, 1969; Indian Hemp Drugs Commission, 1894). The British government chose not to outlaw cultivation and commerce of the herb after ascertaining that it had negligible adverse effects on health, even in chronic application.

Similar conclusions were obtained in the "LaGuardia Report" of 1944 (New York, NY), Mayor's committee on marihuana (Wallace and Cunningham, 1944), which was the first to employ clinical and scientific methods of analysis.

Three important systematic epidemiological studies undertaken by research teams in the 1970s exhaustively examined medical issues in chronic cannabis use, but remain obscure due to limited press runs and out-of-print status. The first of these was *Ganja in Jamaica: A Medical Anthropological Study of Chronic Marihuana Use* (Rubin and Comitas, 1975). Therapeutic claims for cannabis were mentioned, but the focus of study was on "recreational use." Sixty men were included in a hospital study of various clinical parameters if they had maintained a minimum intake of 3 spliffs a day for a minimum of 10 years. Jamaican ganja "spliffs" formed of unfertilized female flowering tops (sinsemilla) tend to be much larger than an American "joint" of 500-1000 mg. The potency of the cannabis was analyzed with measures in 30 samples ranging from 0.7-10.3% THC, with an average of 2.8%.

In 1977, a detailed study was undertaken in Greece, titled *Hashish:Studies of Long-Term Use* (Stefanis, Dornbush and Fink, 1977). Once again 60 subjects smoking for more than 10 years were selected. Hashish potency was 4-5% THC and was generally mixed with tobacco. Alcoholics were excluded.

In 1980, *Cannabis in Costa Rica: A Study of Chronic Marihuana Use* was published (Carter, 1980). Forty-one subjects smoking for 10 years or more were recruited. Although 10 or more cigarettes per day were smoked, the weight of material was only 2 g with an estimated THC range of 24-70 mg per day. Thirteen samples were assayed with a range of 1.27-3.72%, and average of 2.2% THC. Claims of benefit for cough, asthma, headache, hangovers, anorexia, impotence, depression and malaise were mentioned, but once more, the focus was on social use.

The current study is the first designed to examine clinical benefits and side effects of chronic clinical cannabis usage in which known amounts of quality-controlled material has been employed.

A BRIEF HISTORY OF THE COMPASSIONATE IND

Robert Randall was diagnosed with severe glaucoma at age 24 and was expected to become totally blind long before he turned 30. He soon began a fascinating medical odyssey that has been memorialized in his "personal reflection" co-authored by his wife, Alice O'Leary, titled *Marijuana Rx: The Patients' Fight for Medicinal Pot* (Randall and O'Leary, 1998), and other books (Randall, 1991a; Randall, 1991b). Until the day he died on June 2, 2001 at age 52 of complications of AIDS, Randall retained his vision, and remained a vocal advocate for the benefits of clinical cannabis.

His own journey commenced when he independently discovered that smoking a certain amount of cannabis eliminated the annoying visual haloes produced by his glaucoma. A subsequent arrest in August 1975 for cannabis cultivation led in turn to his dogged pursuit of the right to a legal means to supply his medicine of choice. He subsequently learned of medical support for his treatment (Hepler and Frank, 1971). D. Pate has published two more recent reviews (Pate, 1999; Pate, 2001).

Through painstaking documentation and experimentation, Randall subsequently confirmed the inability of medical science to control his intraocular pressure (IOP) by any legal pharmaceutical means. In contrast, smoked cannabis in large and frequent amounts was successful, where even pure THC was not. As Dr. Hepler observed in their experiments together (Randall and O'Leary, 1998, p. 60), "...clearly, something other than THC or in addition to THC is helping to lower your pressures... It seems that marijuana works very, very well."

After a great deal of bureaucratic wrangling, Randall obtained his first government supplied cannabis in November 1976, and the legal case against him was subsequently dismissed. The material he received from his study physician was cultivated in a 5-acre plot at the University of Mississippi, mostly from seeds of Mexican origin, and was rolled and packaged at the Research Triangle Institute in North Carolina under the supervision of the National Institute on Drug Abuse (NIDA).

Randall was encouraged to be thankful, but silent, about his treatment. Instead, he chose a different path (Randall and O'Leary, 1998, p. 134), "Having won, why go mum? There were souls to save. Better to trust my fellow citizens and shout in to the darkness than rely on a devious government dedicated to a fraudulent prohibition." He chose to make it his mission to seek approval of clinical cannabis for other patients.

He developed protocols for glaucoma, multiple sclerosis, chronic pain, and AIDS that he shared with prospective medical marijuana candidates. Randall proved to be a tireless and persistent researcher, ferreting out hidden facts useful to his cause. Through the Freedom of Information Act (FOIA), he discovered in 1978 that the government's cost of cannabis cultivation and production was 90 cents per ounce (28 g), with 2/3 of this cost attributable to security measures. Thus, the actual cost of production approximated 1 cent per gram (US $0.01/g).

Supply and quality control issues arose frequently, and Randall and other patients experienced delays in receipt of shipments or substitution of weaker strains that required doubling of smoked intake.

The AIDS epidemic and its subsequent involvement in the medical marijuana issue suddenly provided an unlimited supply of available patients for the Compassionate IND program, and Randall assisted them as well. Some succumbed before their supply was approved, or shortly thereafter. By 1991, 34 patients were enrolled in the program according to Randall (Randall and O'Leary, 1998), while other sources cite the number as only 15. Facing an onslaught of new applications, the Public Health Service (PHS) in the Bush administration closed the program to new patients in March 1992. A significant number had received medical approval but were never supplied. Randall sought to ascertain who signed the ultimate termination order through the FOIA, but was never successful in this endeavor. At the time of this writing, 7 patients survive in the program.

METHODS
The identities of 6 of 8 of the original Compassionate IND program subjects were known to Patients Out of Time and were contacted in relation to participating in a study of the clinical parameters cited as concerns with chronic cannabis usage. Four subjects agreed to participate, and 3 traveled to Missoula, MT for testing at Montana Neurobehavioral Specialists, and Saint Patrick Hospital on May 3-4, 2001. One patient was tested to the extent possible in her local area due to physical limitations on travel (Patient Demographics: Table 1). Tests included the following (Tests Performed: Table 2): MRI scans of the brain, pulmonary function tests (spirometry), chest X-ray (P-A and lateral), neuropsychological test battery, hormone and immunological assays (CD4 counts), electroencephalography (EEG), P300 testing (a computerized EEG test of memory), and neurological history and clinical examination.

Past medical records were reviewed insofar as possible and the histories were supplemented with additional information. All patients signed informed consent documents, and the St. Patrick Hospital/Community Hospital Joint Investigational Review Board (IRB) reviewed the protocol.

RESULTS AND DISCUSSION
Case Histories and Test Data on Four Compassionate IND Program Patients
In the following section case histories, clinical examinations and objective test results are presented.

Patient A

Medical History: This almost 62-year-old female was born with congenital cataracts in Cali, Colombia and spent 13 years of her life there. There was a question of possible maternal exposure to malaria or quinine. Over time the patient required a series of 11 surgeries on the right eye and 3 on the left for the cataracts and had resulting problems with glaucoma. Her last surgery was complicated by hemorrhaging, leading to immediate and complete loss of vision OD.

By 1976, the patient's intraocular pressure was out of control with all available drugs, many of which caused significant side effects. At that time she started eating and smoking cannabis to treat the condition. She underwent extensive testing in that regard, measuring pressures to titrate the dosage of cannabis. She initially had personal issues with the concept of smoking. Without cannabis her intraocular pressures may run into the 50s, while with it, values are in the teens to 20s. In 1988, she was arrested for cultivation of 6 cannabis plants. Her ophthalmologist noted (Randall and O'Leary, 1998, p. 303), "it's quite clear-cut this is the only thing that will help her." At her trial, she stated in her own defense (Randall and O'Leary, 1998, p. 305), "Marijuana saved my sight. I don't think the law has the right to demand blindness from a citizen."

She was acquitted on the basis of "medical necessity," but her approval for the Compassionate IND program took 6 months. She had smoked cannabis on her own from black market sources for 12 years previously.

At present, she also uses Timoptic® (timolol, beta-blocker) eye drops daily in the morning, but has concerns about resulting bronchoconstriction. She normally uses cannabis 3-4 grams smoked and 3-4 grams orally per day. She feels that the amount that she receives legally from NIDA is insufficient for her medical needs. At times she accepts donations from cannabis buyers' clubs. She admits that the results of these outside cannabis samples on her intraocular pressure are unclear. She has had occasion to go to Amsterdam where intraocular pressures were measured in the teens simply employing cannabis available there. She has used Marinol® on an emergency basis, such as on traveling to Canada, in doses of up to 5-10 mg qid. She reports that it lowers intraocular pressure for one day, but within 3-5 days becomes useless for that purpose.

The patient has a history of cigarette smoking as well, 1-2 packs a day. She quit in 1997, but subsequently went on a "binge" of cigarette smoking for 13 months, finally quitting on New Year's Day 2001. She feels that past pulmonary function has been normal.

She also notes lifelong insomnia that is alleviated by eating cannabis. Without such treatment, she feels she would sleep 4 hours, whereas with it she sleeps 6-7.

She also feels that the drug produces antidepressant and anti-anxiety effects for her. She has a history of scoliosis, but notes no symptoms from this and feels that muscle relaxant effects of cannabis have made her quite limber.

The patient had a history of delirium associated with malaria as a child. She had some hardware in her foot from a 1980 surgery after a fall from platform shoes. She had a hysterectomy for fibroids. The patient was menopausal at age 48 and has had no hormone replacement treatment.

There is no known history of specific meningitis, encephalitis, head trauma, seizures, diabetes, or thyroid problems. She is on no medicine save for cannabis and timolol eye drops. There are allergies to penicillin and tetracycline. She completed the equivalent of high school, and is right handed.

Family history is largely negative, although her 2 children had some cataract involvement. Social history revealed that the patient has worked in the past as a switchboard operator. She is currently disabled due to legal blindness from her condition. She supports herself on Social Security Disability Income (SSDI). She has been an activist with respect to clinical cannabis.

The patient drinks alcohol at a rate of about a bottle of wine a week. She had past heavy use of caffeine, but now drinks decaf only. The patient walks for exercise about an hour a day.

Medical Test Results: Objective: Weight: 132 lbs. OFC (Occipito-frontal Circumference): 55.5 cm. BP: 104/62. General: Very pleasant, cooperative 62-year-old female. Head: normocephalic without bruits. ENT: noteworthy as below. Neck: supple. Carotids: full. Cor: S1, S2 without murmur. On auscultation of the chest, there seemed to be a pro-longed expiratory phase, but no wheezing. Mental Status: The patient was alert and fully oriented. Fund of knowledge, right-left orientation, praxis and naming skills were normal. She was unable to read a grade 6 paragraph with large type due to visual blurring. When it was read to her, memory of the contents was within normal limits. She performed serial 3's well. She remembered 3 objects for 5 minutes. On a word list task she named 15 animals in 30 seconds (normal 10-12). Speech and affect were normal.

Cranial Nerves: I: intact to coconut scent. II: acuity had recently been measured. There was no vision OD, 20/200 OS corrected. Visual fields OS intact to confrontation. Optokinetic nystagmus (OKNs) was present in that eye in all fields. The patient is aphakic with an irregular eccentric pupil OS and clouding OD. The disk on the left appeared normal. There was prominent horizontal nystagmus resembling a congenital pattern. External extraocular movements were normal. Remaining cranial nerves V and VII-XII appeared intact in full.

Motor: The patient had normal tone and strength with no drift. Sensation was intact to fine touch, sharp/dull, vibration, position and graphesthesia. Romberg was negative. The patient performed finger-to-nose and heel-to-shin well. Rapid alternating movements of the hands were slightly clumsy and fine finger movements slightly deliberate. Gait including toe and heel were normal with tandem gait normal, but very carefully done. Reflexes were 2-3+, symmetric with downgoing toes.

The patient underwent a battery of tests. On pulmonary function tests (Table 3), a Functional Vital Capacity (FVC) was 103% predicted. Forced Expiratory Volume in 1 second (FEV 1) was 84% of predicted and the FEV 1/FVC ratio was 0.67. This was read as showing a mild obstructive defect based on the above ratio and flow volume curve morphology.

No restrictive abnormality was noted. A CBC was wholly within normal limits (Table 4). Absolute lymphocyte count was 4.0, CD4 61.6% and absolute CD4 count 2465, all within normal limits. A full endocrine battery was performed (Table 5), including FSH, LH, prolactin, estradiol, estrone, estrogen, testosterone, and progesterone, all within normal limits for age and gender. An EEG was performed during wakefulness and early stages of sleep (read by EBR). A normal alpha background was identifiable at 12 hertz, along with a great deal of beta activity. Occasional left frontal phase reversing sharp waves were seen with rare episodes of slight slowing in the same area. The patient had a P300 test performed with a latency of 355 milliseconds, within normal limits for a normed population in this laboratory. The patient had an MRI brain study without contrast. This was read as showing a mild, symmetric, age consistent cerebral atrophy.

A small focus of T2 hyperintensity and increased signal was noted on the FLAIR sequence in the midpons to the left of midline with no surrounding mass effect or edema. This was felt to be a nonspecific finding representing gliosis most likely from microvascular ischemic change. No corresponding signal abnormality was seen in the same area on a diffusion-weighted sequence. A chest x-ray showed slight hyperinflation of the lung fields with no other findings.

Patient A was very pleasant and cooperative throughout the neuropsychological assessment and appeared to put forth very good effort. She did have very significant visual deficits and as a result, several instruments were dropped from the battery, including Grooved Peg Board, Picture Arrangement, Symbol Search, and the Faces and Family Pictures Subtests from the Wechsler Memory Scale–3rd Edition (WMS-III).

She was able to complete the Trail-Making Test A & B from the Halstead-Reitan Neuropsychological Battery, Spatial Span from the Wechsler Memory Scale–3rd

Edition (WMS-III), and the Wechsler Adult Intelligence Scale–3rd Edition (WAIS-III)-Picture Completion, Digit Symbol, and Matrix Reasoning, but these were not used in interpretation secondary to the very probable interfering effects of her limited sight.

Review of the WAIS-III revealed a Verbal IQ in the upper end of the Average Range (VIQ = 108), and a Performance IQ in the Extremely Low Range, at only the 2nd percentile (PIQ = 69). This latter, however, is secondary to visual deficits as she had extremely low scores on the Digit Symbol and Picture Completion subtests. She obtained an age scaled score of 7 on Block Design; this performance was also adversely impacted by her visual defects to a mild degree.

Assessment of attention and concentration revealed that these abilities are mildly-to-moderately impaired relative to age-matched controls. She demonstrated an abnormally high number of omission errors on the Conner's Continuous Performance Test–2nd Edition (CPT-II) as well as significant variability of reaction time.

Formal assessment of learning and memory revealed that this subject's ability to acquire new verbal material on the WMS-III is within the Average Range relative to age-matched peers. Her Auditory Immediate Index score was in the average range as was her Auditory Delayed Index. She obtained index scores of 97 and 108 on these two indices, respectively. Recognition memory for auditory material was actually in the High Average range, the 75th percentile (Index Score = 110). In contrast she did much more poorly on visual measures secondary to very significant visual defects.

On the California Verbal Learning Test (CVLT), the subject generally performed within normal limits. Although initial learning trials were two standard deviations below expected limits, her ultimate acquisition at Trial 5 was one standard deviation above normative data sets. Short Delay Free Recall was perfectly normal and long delay recall was only one standard deviation below expected levels. This loss of recalled items from short delay to long delay free recall represented a loss that is approximately 1 standard deviation more than expected. Thus, she appeared to have mild difficulties with initial acquisition of very complex verbal material and also appeared to have minimal-to-mild difficulty retaining it in memory relative to age-matched peers. Higher-level executive functions appear to be entirely normal in this patient. The Wisconsin Card Sorting Test (WCST) yielded a T-score of 63, while she obtained a T-score of 42 on the Category Test. Thus, she is still within the parameters seen in a normative data set of age and education-matched peers.

This subject's performance on the Thurstone Word Fluency Test was also entirely normal with a T-score of 51. Likewise, on the Controlled Oral Word Association

Test, she obtained an overall score placing her at the 78th percentile. She produced 26 items on the Animal Naming Test over a 60-second period. This is within normal limits. On the Beck Depression Inventory–2nd Edition, she obtained an overall score of 6, arguing against significant depressive symptoms.

In summary, Patient A appears to have mild-to-moderate difficulty with attention and concentration, and minimal-to-mild difficulty with the acquisition and storage of very complex new verbal material. General learning, however, as measured on the Wechsler Memory Scale–3rd Edition (WMS-III) appears to be within normal limits. Higher-level executive functions and verbal fluency abilities are well within normal limits.

Patient B

Medical History: This 50-year-old white male carries the diagnosis of the nail-patella syndrome, also known as hereditary osteoonychodysplasia, a rare genetic disorder producing hypoplastic nails and kneecaps and renal insufficiency. Information was obtained from the patient, a published affidavit (Randall 1991b), and submitted medical records.

He first smoked cannabis in 1970, but did not become "high." Rather, he felt more relaxed, without his customary muscle spasms and pain. He first actually used clinical cannabis in a different manner. At the time he was mining, and he developed chemical burns in his hands. A Mexican lady gave him a tincture of cannabis flowering tops in grain alcohol to apply. This reduced his hand swelling and burning.

He has been smoking cannabis regularly for medical purposes since about 1974. During a medical crisis in 1985, he suffered a decrease in supply of available cannabis. His recollection is that all the various analgesics he received during this time were ineffective and produced dangerous side effects including sedation and incapacity.

By 1988, he pursued regular usage of cannabis, about 1/8 of an ounce (3½-4 g/d) a day when available. He initiated inquiries with the FDA to obtain legal cannabis. Ultimately, with the assistance of Robert Randall, he received approval from the government in March 1990.

He related a history of deformities from birth including missing fingernails, loose finger joints, and small patellae. He was frequently ill as a child, and at age 10, suffered a progression from conjunctivitis to varicella, strep throat and rheumatic fever. He was hospitalized for 6 months, and required another 3 months of bed rest. Subsequently, he underwent four right knee surgeries, reconstructions and rotations, including 3 arthroscopies. He had had a right wrist graft with non-fusion. He had had right elbow surgery and had a "nicked" ulnar nerve. In the late 1960s he developed both hepatitis A and B with prolonged hospitalizations. Despite this, he pursued heavy manual labor in mining, construction, auto bodywork and aircraft repair. He lost all his teeth by the age of 21. In 1972 he dislocated his knee and had 3 subsequent surgeries. In 1976 he had a wrist fracture with subsequent surgery and later fusion. In 1978 he was hospitalized after a nail wound in his foot failed to heal. In 1983, he injured his back in a fall. Pain continued.

After a 1985 chiropractic session, he became acutely ill with severe back pain. He was given narcotics, and suffered renal failure. He was transferred to a university center. Lithotripsy sessions were followed by transurethral procedures in attempts to clear his nephrolithiasis. Eventually an open procedure was performed for perinephric abscess, but the flank wound failed to heal over the course of a year. Ultimately, it was determined that he was suffering a tubercular nephritis. He took triple therapy with isoniazid (INH), rifampin and pyridoxine regularly for 18 months. Eventually, a massive debridement was necessary, before the flank wound eventually healed. His prolonged convalescence forced him to close his business.

On September 3, 1987, he complained of persistent flank pain and low back discomfort increasing over the preceding 2 years treated with multiple modalities, including TENS unit. He also was using an abdominal binder. Pain radiated to the buttocks and posterior thighs. X rays of the lumbar spine showed spondylolisthesis grade 1 in the lumbar area with no significant motion of flexion extension views.

On April 8, 1988, the patient was seen for right knee pain after a twisting injury and fall. An effusion developed. X rays showed a micropatella consistent with nail-patella syndrome, but no evidence of fracture. He was treated conservatively. In October, 1988, chest x-ray showed a diffuse nodular infiltrate unchanged since September 1985.

By June 7, 1989, the patient was in a wheelchair, but was able to ambulate with a cane. Previous X rays showed bilateral iliac spurs. His chart notes included an FDA consent form in relation to the patient's use of cannabis (Figure 2). On subsequent visits, he had been approved for the Compassionate IND program, and was smoking 10 cannabis cigarettes a day.

On April 1, 1991, some cough was noted attributed to cigarettes. As a baseline, very severe pain was noted in the extremities, but this was reduced to slight to moderate on subsequent visits. By April 17, 1991, the patient was on no medicines except for cannabis. By January 18, 1993, he was said to have only slight to moderate problems with a cane for support. There were some abdominal spasms.

On the May 14, 1996 visit, he was smoking 10 cannabis cigarettes a day. He used occasional aspirin for increased pain. He had resumed smoking ½ to 1 pack of cigarettes a day. Examination was fairly unremarkable save for orthopedic deformities. He was able to walk on his toes and heels. The patient was given 2 more packages of 300 marijuana cigarettes.

On July 16, 1996, the patient was seen for disability examination. It was noted the patient had suffered for many years from lack of strength, mobility and range of motion, and persistent episodes of nausea and muscle spasms. The note indicated, "the marijuana helps the patient function better in the sense that he has increased flexibility, increased strength and range of motion. He has less nausea and less muscle spasm." He needed to shift into different positions at home to get comfortable and could do a sit down type job for an hour or two at most before experiencing spasms, pain and nausea. He had limited backward flexion, and limited right hand strength. He was unable to kneel. He could walk 50 feet before needing to rest, used a cane and sometimes a wheelchair for longer distances. It was felt he could not be a traveling salesman, and any prospective job would require frequent rests. Overall, he was assessed as having a significant functional impairment due to nail-patella syndrome, and was judged unemployable in the short or long term, with little rehabilitation potential.

A May 9, 1997 letter indicates, "continues to smoke about 8-10 marijuana cigarettes per day and still continues to benefit from that medication. He has less pain, less spasms, he is able to ambulate better. His nausea is improved, he is able to sleep better. He is making some slow deterioration of this disease process." It goes on to say, "I personally do feel that [Patient B] continues to benefit from marijuana and hope that we can continue providing this unfortunate man with marijuana medication."

On May 10, 2000, a letter to FDA noted the patient continued to do well on the therapy, smoking 8-10 cigarettes per day without other medication. He continued to function well using a cane and occasionally a wheelchair when bothered by spasms and nausea.

At present, he utilizes about 7 grams a day or ¼ ounce of NIDA material that is 3.75% THC, and was processed in April 1999. The patient cleans the cannabis to a minimal degree first, estimating a loss of about 25% of material. He indicates that he has been short on his supply 3 times in 10 years, generally for 1-2 weeks, secondary to lack of supply or paperwork problems. When this occurs he suffers more nausea and muscle spasms and is less active as a consequence. He was never allowed to try Marinol®, and points out that he could not afford it in any event.

The patient reports continued problems with pain in the back, hips and legs, also in the upper extremities, right greater than left. When he undergoes spasms the pain rises to a 10 on a 10-point scale and is associated with projectile emesis. His baseline level of pain is 6-7/10. He notes that this pain was never helped by prescription medicines. Morphine sulfate produced a minimal decrement in pain for up to two hours, but caused inebriation. By the third day of application it would become totally ineffective. Without cannabis he feels that he would need very high doses of narcotics. Eventually he had become allergic to most pharmaceutical preparations, or had side effects of nausea. The latter continues, particularly in static positions, which without cannabis treatment he rates as a 10/10. In 1985, he was without cannabis for some 30 days and lost 57 pounds when his supply ran out at the same time that he had TB nephritis. In relation to the spasms, these can occur anywhere in his body. He feels the medicine eliminates them or substantially reduces nocturnal manifestations. Without it he would be "running" at night.

He has no history of diabetes, thyroid problems, meningitis, encephalitis, or head trauma. He may have had seizures associated with fever. The patient has taken rare antibiotics for staph infections of the skin. He feels that he has had lots of reactions to synthetic chemicals of various types, which he considers quite serious. The patient left school at age 14 originally, but attained a GED and had some junior college experience.

He is left-handed.

Family history is noteworthy for nail-patella syndrome in mother, niece, two sisters, nephew and daughter. One sister died of the disease at age 44. He has two unaffected children. His affected daughter does not receive legal cannabis. His father died of TB and tumors at age 40.

Social History: He currently smokes cigarettes about ½ pack a day, but as high as a pack a day in the past. The patient drinks beer about 1 a month, with little alcohol use in 10 years. The patient last worked full-time in 1985, and part-time in 1990. He is on SSDI, but does volunteer and activist work. The patient is able to walk very little due to pain, but bikes when he can, a short distance. The patient sleeps from 10 p.m. to 6 a.m., but this is disrupted due to pain or nausea.

Medical Test Results: Weight: 173 lbs. Height: 69 inches (BMI: 25.6). OFC: 60 cm. BP: 122/80. General: Very pleasant, cooperative 50 YOM who appears somewhat wizened. Head: normocephalic without bruits. ENT was noteworthy for edentulous state. Neck: supple. Carotids: full, without bruit. Cor: S1, S2 without murmur. The patient has a large indentation scar in the right flank. Palpation to the spine was un-remarkable. Chest auscultation revealed a prolonged expiratory phase without wheezing. Abdominal examination was unremarkable. He had dysplastic nails.

Mental Status: The patient was alert and fully oriented. Fund of knowledge, right-left orientation, praxis and naming skills were normal. He read a grade 6 paragraph well with good recall. Serial 3's were well done. Signature was normal. He remembered 2 of 3 objects after 5 minutes with hesitation, failed the third with hint, but got it with choice of 3. He had a hoarse voice. He named 11 animals in 30 seconds (normal). Affect was normal. Cranial Nerves: I: intact. II: acuity was measured as 20/25 OD, 20/50 OS uncorrected. Fields and OKNs were normal. Fundi were benign. Pupils equally reactive with full EOMs and no nystagmus. Remaining cranial nerves V and VII-XII were unremarkable.

On motor examination, the patient had hypotonicity, but decreased bulk. The patient lacked full elbow extension on the right. His strength was generally 4+ secondary to limitations and pain. There was no arm drift. Sensation was intact to fine touch, vibration, position and graphesthesia, but there was some slight vibratory loss in the feet. Romberg was negative. The patient performed finger-to-nose well. Heel-to-shin required partial assist of the hands. Rapid alternating movements of the hands were very slow on the right secondary to mechanical problems. Fine finger movements were normal. The patient had a stiff, bent gait, but toe gait appeared more normal. On heel gait he favored the left leg. Tandem gait was difficult due to back pain and he wavered some. I was unable to ascertain reflexes at the biceps on the right, but responses elsewhere were 1-2+ with downgoing toes.

The patient underwent the prescribed battery of tests. Pulmonary function tests revealed an FVC of 107% of predicted, FEV 1 of 95% of predicted, and FEV 1/FVC of 0.75. This was interpreted as within normal limits, but with a slightly prolonged forced expiratory time. Acomplete blood count showed some mild polycythemia, probably due to tobacco smoking. An absolute lymphocyte count was 3.4 with CD4 count 68.7% and absolute count of 2324. The patient had a full endocrine battery. Measurement of FSH, LH, prolactin, estradiol, estrone, estrogen, testosterone and progesterone were wholly within normal limits for age and gender. An EEG was performed during wakefulness and was within normal limits, but did demonstrate some low voltage fast activity in the beta range, with no focal or epileptiform activity. The patient had a P300 response with a latency of 338 milliseconds, within normal limits for the laboratory. An MRI of the brain without contrast was read as normal. A PA and lateral chest was read as normal.

Patient B was friendly and cooperative and appeared to put forth very good effort on neuropsychological testing. On the WAIS-III, he obtained Verbal and Performance IQ Scores in the Average Range (VIQ = 105 and PIQ = 92). In terms of overall intellectual functioning, he obtained an overall score placing him at the 50th percentile (Full Scale IQ = 100). Assessment of attention and concentration with the CPT-II revealed that these abilities tended toward mildly-to-moderately impaired relative to the normative data set. He made an abnormally high number of omission errors and also demonstrated substantial variability in his reaction time. He also became more variable as time progressed over this 14-minute measure.

On the WMS-III, he obtained Auditory Immediate and Auditory Delayed Index scores of 89 and 86, placing him in the low average range. His Auditory Recognition Delayed Index was in the average range with an index score of 90. Visual Immediate and Visual Delayed abilities were also in the low average range with index scores of 88 on both. Overall, these performances are within normal limits, albeit it in the low average range.

On the CVLT, this patient's initial acquisition of items after the first trial was one standard deviation below expected levels, and his recall after five learning trials was two standard deviations below. Short Delay Free Recall and Long Delay Free Recall were essentially at the same level. Thus, his acquisition of very complex verbal material does appear at least mildly impaired. Interestingly, he does not lose this information from memory after a delay.

Assessment of higher-level executive functions yields an overall performance on the WCST at a mildly impaired level relative to age and education matched peers, with a T-score of 38. His overall performance on the Category Test was in the borderline range with a T-score of 40. He also had difficulty following new complex sequences with a T-score of 40 on the Trails A Subtest and a T-score of 32 (mildly-to-moderately impaired) on the Trails B component.

Simple motor testing reveals that Tapping Speed was within normal limits, but he had difficulty with fine motor coordination on the Groove Pegboard Test with his dominant left hand. He obtained a T-score of 36 on this particular measure with his left hand, a T-score of 42 with his right hand.

On the Thurstone Word Fluency Test, he obtained a T-score of 54 and a T-score of 40.2 on the Controlled Oral Word Association Test. Animal naming was within normal limits with a total score of 22.

In summary, Patient B does appear to have a mild-to-moderate impairment of attention and concentration, and his ability to acquire new, complex detailed verbal material also appears to be mildly-to-moderately impaired. There is quite some variability in this regard, however, with performances on the Wechsler Memory Scale–3rd Edition (WMS-III) being generally within normal limits, and his California Verbal Learning Test (CVLT) performance falling approximately 2 standard deviations below expected levels. He had difficulty on motor tasks. His performances may have been adversely affected by peripheral pain as he complained of such during the assessment process. His overall score of 0 on the Beck Depression Inventory (BDI) argues against significant depressive symptoms.

Patient C

Medical History: This 48-year-old male carries a diagnosis of multiple congenital cartilaginous exostoses, an autosomal dominant disorder. History was obtained from the patient, a published affidavit (Randall, 1991b), and submitted progress notes dating from December 5, 1996.

He recalls few medical problems until age 10, when he threw a baseball and his arm became paralyzed for a few hours. Radiographs revealed what was interpreted as an old fracture that had healed with jagged bone fragments. Multiple referrals ensued, and ultimately 250 bony tumors were found throughout his body. He was diagnosed as having multiple congenital cartilaginous exostoses. Each was capable of growth, massive tissue disruption, pain, and malignant transformation.

By age 17, he underwent multiple surgical procedures on the left leg, and right wrist. By age 12, constant pain and frequent hemorrhages severely limited his gait along with other basic functions. He required a home tutor by grade 7. By age 14, he required ongoing narcotics for analgesia, escalating to Dilaudid® (hydromorphone), and Sopor® (methaqualone, now Schedule I in USA) for sleep. He reports resultant fatigue, ennui, and disorientation as side effects.

At age 20, he developed a large bone spur on the right ankle, which recurred dramatically after one surgery. Amputation was recommended, but refused. At age 22, a fist-sized tumor was removed from the pelvis. A medical odyssey ensued, which failed to identify better therapies and he required massive doses of hydromorphone, methaqualone, and muscle relaxants.

He described himself as a conservative young man who was against drugs, but in college acquiesced to try marijuana. He enjoyed chess, but was normally able to sit for only 5-10 minutes without pain. One day, he smoked cannabis and an hour into a chess match he remained pain-free.

After discussion with his doctor, he experimented by smoking it regularly for 6 months. He noted a marked enhancement of his analgesia, and a reduction on his dependence on hydromorphone (taken intravenously for some time), Demerol® (meperidine), and hypnotics. Cannabis analgesia exceeded that of any prescription drugs.

He began to investigate possible legal avenues to obtain cannabis, and met Robert Randall in 1978. By 1979, he was spending $3000 annually on therapeutic cannabis through the black market, an unsustainable burden. A Byzantine bureaucratic process ensued over several years, with final FDA approval of his IND application in November 1982. Weekly monitoring sessions including needle electromyography (EMG) were deemed necessary to assess the effects of treatment in his protocol. Subsequently, he described numerous instances of delayed shipments of cannabis, or exhaustion of supplies of higher potency product. Substitution of 1% THC cannabis required a doubling of dosage to 20 cannabis joints a day.

He was once arrested in Florida despite documentation, handcuffed and jailed overnight, sustaining an ankle hemorrhage in the process. Only 4 of 7 confiscated joints were ultimately returned. Beyond this, he describes cannabis as much safer than prescribed medicine, and free of serious adverse effects except chest pain with prolonged usage of inferior product.

In 1992, Patient C had occasion to try Marinol® during a stockholders meeting in Canada due to his legal proscription from traveling with cannabis. Although he had no side effects on a dose of 10 mg, it was without any benefits, and left his muscles very tight and painful.

Detailed progress notes from the last several years were obtained and will be summarized. December 5, 1996, the patient was using 10-20 mg of baclofen and 10-15 cannabis cigarettes a day. Assessment was of multiple congenital cartilaginous exostoses with hepatitis C, and GE re-flux. He was prescribed diazepam 5 mg for spasm. An EKG was read as showing normal sinus rhythm. February 28, 1996, the patient had pulmonary functions with FVC 112% of predicted, FEV 1 of 79% of predicted, read as indicating mild obstruction. January 24, 1997, he had episodic spasm with pain affecting both arms and legs. It was noted at the time that the patient had a malunion of the right radius. He was down to 2-3 cannabis cigarettes a day, as he had received no supply from NIDA since September 1996, due to logistical problems in seeing his study physician. A transfer of providers was recommended. September 4, 1997, he remained on baclofen 10 mg p.m., 5 mg a.m. and Prilosec® (omeprazole) for epigastric discomfort that had been going on for 7 years, and cannabis 12 cigarettes a day. September 9, 1997, the patient had a chest x-ray with no findings. September 9, 1997, the patient had laboratory tests done, including a CBC, non-reactive hepatitis A and B tests, and normal thyroid functions. Glucose was low at 24, potassium high at 5.4, SGOT 79 with other parameters negative. September 17, 1997, the patient was said to be doing well smoking 10-12 cannabis cigarettes a day with dramatic decreases in frequency and intensity of flexor spasms. He was also taking baclofen. It was noted that with strong spasms the patient would bruise his skin and sometimes even bleed. His weight was constant, appetite normal. Neurological exam was fairly unremarkable. He was asked to slowly decrease the baclofen to 2.5 mg bid. May 13, 1998, the patient was said to be doing quite well. In the interim, a liver biopsy demonstrated minimal changes secondary to hepatitis C. Chest X rays were said to show no changes. The prior December the patient had twisted his left knee with a lot of swelling, and an MRI revealed a minor crack in the tibial head. Pain was under good control with 12 cannabis cigarettes a day with only occasional muscle spasms. Exam was unremarkable. He was said to be doing quite well off of the baclofen and was asked to continue 12 cigarettes of cannabis a day. May 26, 1999, the patient related no difficulty breathing. Weight was constant. There was dull pain in the ankles and some sharp shooting also in the knees. There was minor weakness in the right hand with no other deficits. The remainder of the exam was normal. The patient was felt to be doing well and advised to continue 12 cannabis cigarettes a day. October 6, 1999, the patient was seen in follow up, was on omeprazole, Vitamin C, and cannabis. The patient had some congestion and mildly productive cough. He was felt to have acute bronchitis and was given cough syrup. January 5, 2000, the patient had pulmonary functions done with an FVC 118% of predicted, FEV 1 82% of predicted. This was felt to indicate borderline obstruction. January 13, 2000, glucose was 126, BUN 26, SGOT 71 with other parameters normal, including CBC. Hepatitis C antibody was reactive with other titers negative. Thyroid functions were normal. An SGPT was 181. May 4, 2000, the patient was occasionally playing softball and had no complaints of shortness of breath. Again there was mild weakness of the hand with other muscles normal. It was felt that the patient was doing well without aches, pains or spasms on his cannabis. November 21, 2000, the patient had noticed some increased discomfort following a motor vehicle accident the prior month wherein he was rear-ended and had neck pain. Subsequently, he noted persistent pain in the right thigh. An X ray was negative. He tried physical therapy, heat and electrical stimulation. He noted more muscle tension with weather change. No neurological changes were observed. December 28, 2000, the patient was on his omeprazole and cannabis. January 6, 2001, SGOT was 50, SGPT 94 with normal CBC and PSA. A cholesterol total was 221 with LDL 136.

At the time he was examined in Missoula, he noted constant baseline pain of 9-10 on a 10-point scale without cannabis. At rest, with cannabis this fell to a 4/10. He was smoking 9 grams a day of 2.7% THC NIDA cannabis, or 11 ounces every 25 days. At times he has had to cut back due to an inadequate supply. He would sometimes have to use street cannabis at a cost $110 per quarter ounce (circa $16/g) of an estimated 4-5% THC content. Interestingly, although he found the flavor was an improvement over the government supply, he noted little difference in analgesic effect except for a greater relaxation effect.

Interestingly, even with extensive cannabis use there are only two times he thinks that he ever may have been "high." One time he left his coat somewhere in freezing weather, which is extremely uncharacteristic, and the other he had been without cannabis for a long time and briefly felt euphoric while smoking. However, once he advanced to a second joint, this feeling was gone.

The patient has the most problems with the left arm where pain is a 7-8/10 when there are flare-ups despite medicine. This decreases after he takes rofecoxib (Vioxx®) for a week. He experiences pain in both knees, but usually minimal (1-2/10) with his cannabis. He may periodically pull a muscle or hemorrhage, especially in the ribs. He has occasional problems in the wrist.

The patient's sleep remains disrupted rarely attaining 6 hours total. Typically, he is up every 45 to 60 minutes with stiffness and needs to have pillows to position himself. He once got 8 hours of sleep with methaqualone (now illegal in USA), waking only twice.

He feels that his hepatitis C is asymptomatic and was probably due to a transfusion in his teens. Although he did use hydromorphone intravenously for a long period of time, he feels that he pursued a scrupulous aseptic technique. Besides surgeries noted above, he has dental caps due to bruxism, and tonsillectomy. He has had past hypertension, which he feels was work related. There is no history of diabetes, thyroid problems, meningitis, encephalitis, head trauma or seizures. He uses only omeprazole 30 mg a day regularly in addition to his cannabis. He is allergic to barbiturates. The patient had 3 semesters of college. He is primarily right-handed, somewhat ambidextrous.

Family history is negative for other known involvement, but his father was adopted. His mother has migraine.

Social History: The patient works full time as a stockbroker. He is also a very decorated disabled sailor. He plays softball once a week. He may use a stationary bike about 10 minutes at a time, but this is subject to weather effects. He does not smoke tobacco. The patient drinks about 1.75 liters of Jack Daniels whiskey every 10-14 days, which helps him sleep. He does not drink coffee.

Medical Test Results: Weight: 153 lbs. Height: 5ft 4½in. General: Very pleasant, cooperative 48-year-old white male who is somewhat obese (BMI: 25.5). Head: normocephalic without bruits. ENT: unre-markable. Neck: supple. Carotids: full, without bruits. Cor: S1, S2 without murmur. The patient had very slight gynecomastia. He has prominent exostoses of the left shoulder, left wrist, right shoulder, and right calf.

Auscultation of the chest revealed a prolonged expiratory phase without wheezing. Abdominal palpation was negative.

Mental Status: The patient was alert and fully oriented. He knew the president and had normal right-left orientation, praxis and naming skills. He read a grade 6 paragraph well with good recall. Serial 3's were done very rapidly. He remembered 3 objects for 5 minutes. He named 15 animals in 30 seconds, which is well above the average of 10-12.

Speech and affect were normal.

Cranial Nerves: I: intact. II: fields and OKNs were normal. Fundi were benign. Pupils were equally reactive with full EOMs and no nystagmus. Remaining cranial nerves V and VII-XII were unremarkable. On motor exam, the patient had some limitation due to pain, but seemed to have good strength throughout except for 4+/5 foot dorsiflexion on the right. There was no drift. Sensation was intact to fine touch, vibration, position and graphesthesia, but there was decrease in sharp/dull discrimination at the top of the right foot secondary to post-operative changes. Romberg was negative. Finger-to-nose and rapid alternating movements of the hands were normal. Heel-to-shin was incomplete on the right, better on the left. Fine finger movements were minimally decreased. On gait testing the patient slightly favored the right leg at the ankle. Toe gait looked better. Heel gait was barely possible due to pain on the right side. Tandem gait was minimally hesitant. Reflexes were 1+, symmetric with downgoing toes.

Medical Test Results: On pulmonary function tests, an FVC was 108% of predicted and FEV 1 67% of predicted. A FEV 1/FVC was 0.51 felt to be indicative of a moderate obstructive defect based on the latter ratio and flow volume curve morphology. No restrictive abnormality was noted.

A CBC was wholly within normal limits. An absolute lymphocyte count was 1.8 with CD4 49.1% and CD4 absolute count of 911. An endocrine battery, including FSH, LH, prolactin, estradiol, estrone, estrogen, testosterone and progesterone, was wholly within normal limits for age and gender.

An EEG was performed during wakefulness and early stages of sleep, which was within broad normal limits. There was a good bit of low voltage fast activity in the beta range. No focal nor epileptiform activity was appreciated. A P300 showed a latency of 262 milliseconds felt to be within normal limits for the lab. An MRI was performed without contrast. There was felt to be no definite abnormality of an acute nature. There were some minor changes in the right parietal area suggestive of a mild degree of gliosis with associated dilated perivascular spaces of doubtful significance. There was a small area of abnormal signal in the right parotid gland overlying the right masseter muscle felt to be probably benign.

P-A and lateral chest X rays were taken. These were read as showing a pulmonary nodule in the left upper lobe with minimal airway changes. One examiner (EBR) reviewed those films and felt that the lesion was actually located in a rib. As a result, the patient underwent a CT scan of the chest after returning home. This showed no evidence of mass, lymphadenopathy, or pulmonary nodules. A small amount of pleural calcification was noted. An exostosis was noted in the right anterior 3rd rib, accounting for the false-positive chest X ray.

On neuropsychological testing, Patient C was pleasant, cooperative, and appeared to put forth very good effort. His attention was noted to be quite poor at times and many instructions had to be repeated.

On the WAIS-III, he obtained Verbal and Performance IQ Scores in the Average Range with a Verbal IQ of 103 and a Performance IQ of 104. In terms of overall intellectual functioning, he is currently performing at a level equal to or above 58 percent of the general population (Full Scale IQ = 103).

Assessment of attention and concentration with the CPT-II revealed that immediate attentional abilities were within normal limits. His ability to concentrate, however, did appear mildly impaired, as he tended to lose efficiency with the passage of time. Thus, vigilance appeared to be mildly decreased relative to a normative data set.

On the WMS-III, Patient C obtained an Auditory Immediate Index in the Average Range at the 70th percentile. His Auditory Immediate Index was 108. Auditory Delayed Index was also 108, placing him in the Average Range, and his Auditory Recognition Delayed Index was 115, placing him in the High Average Range. The Visual Immediate Index was 115 with a Visual Delayed Index of 122, performances in the High Average and Superior Ranges, respectively.

On the CVLT, this patient's initial acquisition on Trial One was two standard deviations below expected levels and his acquisition of only ten items by Trial 5 was one standard deviation below expected levels.

Short Delay Free Recall was also one standard deviation below expected levels but he performed within normal limits if provided cues. His ultimate free recall after a 20-minute delay was also one standard deviation below expected levels. There was not a substantial loss of information between Long Delay and Short Delay Free Recall trials. Thus, his ability to acquire very complex and detailed new verbal material does appear minimally-to-mildly decreased relative to age matched peers, well below his ability to acquire new thematically organized verbal material, which was in the above average range. Memory, however, appears normal.

Assessment of higher level executive functions yielded a T-score of 45 on the WCST and a T-score of 44 on the Category Test from the Halstead-Reitan Neuropsychological Battery. His ability to follow new complex sequences was entirely within normal limits as indicated by T-scores of 52 and 62 on Trail Making Test A and B, respectively.

Simple motor speed measured by Finger Tapping was within normal limits, bilaterally, as was fine motor coordination measured by the Grooved Pegboard Test.

His performance on the Thurstone Word Fluency Test yielded a T-score of 56, which is entirely within normal limits relative to age and education-matched peers. Likewise, his overall performance on the Controlled Oral Word Association Test yielded a T-score of 52.52, and Animal Naming Fluency also was within normal limits. His overall score on the Beck Depression Inventory-2nd Edition (BDI-II) was 0.

Overall, Patient C appears to have mild difficulty sustaining attention and also minimal-to-mild difficulty with the acquisition of very new, complex verbal material. Overall, however, he appears to be functioning quite well.

Patient D
Medical History: This 45-year-old female carries a diagnosis of multiple sclerosis (MS). The patient was interviewed by telephone (EBR) in lieu of the possibility of contemporaneous examination. The patient feels her first problem may have occurred at age 18 when her vision sequentially went completely black for two months with slow improvement over a subsequent four months. A possible attribution to oral contraception was hypothesized. She was subsequently evaluated at a quarternary referral center and diagnosed as having retro-bulbar neuritis. She was prescribed nicotinic acid. On re-evaluation in 1983, no active disease was noted. On May 29, 1986, best corrected vision was 20/30 OD, 20/25 OS. By May 19, 1988, values fell to 20/200 OD, and 20/70 OS. The patient was formally diagnosed as having MS April 1 of that year with associated bilateral optic neuropathy. She had had symptoms for perhaps 6 months with blurring in both eyes and leg spasms that interfered with walking. The patient had never used cannabis recreationally, and began it only because of her symptoms.

She has been followed in her local area by a psychiatrist and neurologist. Extensive, well-documented notes commencing December 20, 1989 were provided, and will be summarized. When first seen on that date the patient was married for the second time. It was noted that she had been diagnosed with MS about a year and a half previously and had been on diazepam from time-to-time. She was taking 10 mg tid to cope with stress. She had previously tried trazodone and buspirone, had become paralyzed with her MS, and was consequently very frightened of these medicines. On examination she was felt to be quite anxious and was provisionally diagnosed as having a dysthymic disorder.

On March 20, 1990, she seemed to be suffering from more depression, although she managed to smile. She described difficulty with self-esteem and hopelessness. She had only been taking diazepam intermittently and was rather prescribed Prozac® (fluoxetine) 20 mg and Xanax® (alprazolam) 0.25 mg up to 3 times a day. She was felt to have recurrent major depression. On subsequent visits the patient had slight adjustments of medicine and was feeling better by May 2, 1990. By August 6, 1990, the patient was having greater difficulties with insomnia. She was given trazodone 50 mg at bedtime on a trial basis. August 24, 1990, the patient was only sleeping until 4 a.m., which was about 2 hours better than without medicine. This was increased to 75 mg.

The patient had heard about some studies of using cannabis in MS as a relaxing agent. She indicated that she had tried this with a good relaxation response. There was a discussion of possible effects on the lungs, and her expected diminished life expectancy because of MS. She was given a prescription for Marinol® (dronabinol, synthetic THC) 10 mg to be tried q 4 hours prn to see if this would help with relaxation and nausea.

When seen September 5, 1990, she had found that the Marinol® had reduced the nausea considerably and had even helped her vision. She continued on fluoxetine. September 27, 1990, the patient was not sleeping well, possibly due to fluoxetine, and was given a benzodiazepine. October 17, 1990, the patient was seen in follow up and was on Xanax® (alprazolam). It was noted that she had improvement with Marinol®, but the patient noted she actually had a better response to smoked cannabis. They began to look into obtaining a legal supply. December 3, 1990, the patient reported increased depression and was increased to 40 mg a day of fluoxetine. December 5, 1990, the patient had recurrent depression even on the fluoxetine 2 a day and low dose alprazolam. Apparently, her doctor had received notification that he could no longer prescribe Marinol® "off label" unless a Schedule I permit for cannabis was being pursued. December 19, 1990, the patient reported nausea, for which some of her remaining Marinol® had helped. January 16, 1991, the patient complained of spasticity spells and episodes of nausea. She had run out of Marinol® and had no cannabis supply. She indicated she had tried other medications without success and was resistant to try others due to side effects. February 20, 1991, the patient had purchased illicit cannabis in the interim. April, 16, 1991, the patient continued on fluoxetine 20 mg bid. More jerkiness was noted with increased spasticity. She had not smoked cannabis before coming in. It was felt that she would need 6 cannabis cigarettes a day to reduce symptoms. May 10, 1991, she was taking alprazolam about every 2 weeks. She was continuing to have some spasms. She continued to try cannabis illicitly, but had not yet obtained it legally. June 14, 1991, she had lost her driver's license due to visual problems associated with MS. During this interval there were more marital issues. July 2, 1991, it was indicated the patient was legally blind and there were no possible corrective measures. Plans were in place to obtain legal cannabis for spasticity and nervous problems. It was noted that cannabis seemed to be very effective for her clinically. August 7, 1991, the patient was still without a supply and complained of her legs jerking at night, and increased difficulty walking. The patient requested Marinol®, but this could not be prescribed. She was given baclofen 5 mg tid to try. August 30, 1991, she received her fist shipment of NIDA cannabis, seven months after approval of the Compassionate IND. The patient was advised that she should confine her use to government cannabis. She was having problems with her gait, able to walk only with a cane. There were continued vision problems. She complained of left sided weakness. The patient smoked a cannabis cigarette in front of the doctor, which led to her feeling better. It was suggested she try 3 cannabis cigarettes a day. September 3, 1991, the patient reported that the government supply of cannabis did not have the "punch" that street bought material had. Her dose was increased to 5 joints a day. It was indicated that her spasticity responded positively to the dose increase. September 11, 1991, the patient was on 5 NIDA cigarettes a day. This was helping her spasticity. She was unclear as to whether her vision was helped. September 20, 1991, it was felt that 7 cigarettes a day would be necessary. The patient reported increased muscular activity, uncontrollable at times. October 2, 1991, the patient had run out and was noticeably more spastic on examination. Her dose was increased to 10 a day. October 9, 1991, the patient was on 10 cannabis cigarettes a day of the strongest available dosage, which seemed to help her spasticity. She was walking without a cane. It was not felt that her depression was improved. November 4, 1991, she had been out of her supply for 10 days. Spasticity increased and she complained of pain in the left leg. Increased tone was noted throughout the body. December 5, 1991, apparently a supply came in of lower potency cannabis. December 19, 1991, it was felt she had continued improvement of her spasticity with better gait. February 14, 1992, she was using 1 can of cannabis a month, equal to 300 cigarettes. The patient reported she had not been falling. March 13, 1992, she continued the cannabis at the same rate, plus 40 mg of fluoxetine and no alprazolam. The patient reported she was able to walk, swim better, and do all of her ADL's much easier than she could prior to the cannabis. There was no observable gait disturbance on exam. April 14, 1992, it was felt that she got a lot of relief from her medicine and that it "probably offers her greater efficacy in her spasticity, also, than Valium would." May 19, 1992, the patient continued to be stable with no exacerbations of her MS and the spasticity under good control. There were concerns about periodontal disease from her dentist. It was thought she might do better with less smoking of a higher potency supply. The patient was also smoking cigarettes and was subsequently advised to avoid tobacco. By July 17, 1992 she continued to respond to cannabis. September 18, 1992, reflexes were equal and not hyperactive. November 16, 1992, there was an increase of depression slowly and insidiously. December 9, 1992, the patient had been off of her treatment for a week and was very shaky. Smoking a joint in front of her doctor caused her to become calm, less shaky and better able to walk. January 19, 1993, she got her first cans of the stronger cannabis, which the patient felt more effective after smoking one joint. March 22, 1993, she was smoking 6-7 a day. She seemed better after smoking one in the office. April 22, 1993, the patient was smoking 10 cigarettes a day. Smoking produced a decrease in spasticity as observed. There were no adverse effects that were noted in the office. May 24, 1993, the patient was tried on lorazepam. June 24, 1993, the patient was upset with financial issues and was placed on Mellaril® (thioridazine). July 22, 1993, when she was examined, no tremor or spasticity was noted. Again cannabis was smoked with no adverse effects noted. August 30, 1993, the patient requested a decrease in her fluoxetine. She felt that spasticity and depression were both helped by the cannabis. September 29, 1993, the patient reported that on a lower fluoxetine dose she was getting tearful. Reflexes were not hyperactive. November 2, 1993, the patient had some paresthesias on the left side, but was maintaining good motor control. December 28, 1993, she was tried on bupropion. January 4, 1994, problems had been noted on bupropion and it was not as effective. She was tried on sertraline. She reported that the cannabis helped her to not think about her MS. She was having fewer spasticity problems. February 4, 1994, when the patient smoked cannabis in the office, she seemed to be a little more talkative and relax significantly with less spasticity and no adverse effects. February 28, 1994, again significant relief from spasticity was noted upon smoking. March 30, 1994, the patient had some numbness and tingling in the limbs. The patient reported the new material was stronger and had a better effect. May 9, 1994, some increase in emotional lability was noted. The patient was taken off of sertraline and put on Effexor® (venlafaxine). May 25, 1994, she was unable to tolerate the latter and was started back on fluoxetine. August 29, 1994, she continued on fluoxetine and cannabis. Smoking a joint calmed her and limited tremor. September 28, 1994, it was indicated in relation to cannabis "it seems to have a positive effect on her mental status overall." October 31, 1994, the patient was felt to be without signs of depression. She actually lowered her dose on a higher potency material. February 1, 1995, the patient was on diazepam again. February 14, 1995, she was increasingly shaky and tearful. March 29, 1995, she was hardly able to walk due to an exacerbation. May 2, 1995, she still needed support. At the same time the patient was having marital difficulties. August 4, 1995, the patient reported she could see much better with the cannabis. By September 6, 1995, she was walking quite well and was no longer on diazepam, merely the fluoxetine and cannabis. October 4, 1995, she continued to walk well with no problems. January 17, 1996, an MRI revealed multiple bilateral periventricular and diffuse white matter changes in the cerebrum and cerebellum, but seemingly fewer than on a April 4, 1995 study. April 19, 1996, the patient had been out of cannabis for a week and was experiencing more spasticity and ambulation difficulties. She was more depressed. May 17, 1996, the patient had been tried on a stimulant. July 10, 1996, the patient reported that cannabis was the only thing that had helped her with her symptoms over the course of her illness. By September 25, 1996, the patient had been without medicine for a month and had to buy it on the street. She had lost weight and her condition had reportedly decompensated to some degree. The patient reported a 10-pound weight loss. November 13, 1996, the patient was having difficulty sleeping, but did not wish to take trazodone. November 27, 1996, the patient had fallen and had a brief loss of consciousness. December 5, 1996, she had had an episode of spasticity that was the worse she had ever had, starting in the neck and going down her back. January 8, 1997, cannabis came in after a summer drought since September 25. An emergency supply was requested. January 22, 1997, the patient remained concerned about lack of cannabis supply. February 5, 1997, she continued with this concern. February 19, 1997, there was discussion of difficulty the patient had experienced with the authorities in an airport. April 2, 1997, it was felt the patient continued to get a great deal of relief from smoking 10 joints a day without any adverse effects. July 2, 1997, the patient was observed to become more loquacious and interactive after dosing. Janary 29, 1998, the patient was not complaining of spasticity, seeming to have considerable relief with cannabis. Her fluoxetine was lowered to 20 mg a day. March 24, 1998, it was felt that she had a very slow progression of her MS helped by her consumption of cannabis. September 22, 1998, the patient said that the medicine took away her fear of the disease and when she would get a pain she would be able to smoke and take it away. October 27, 1998, she apparently had been out of her supply for 6 weeks, but had gotten by smoking only 4 cigarettes a day instead of the usual 10. January 24, 1998, the patient was doing relatively well and was walking with a cane. December 22, 1998, she was having increasing problems. January 26, 1999, the patient indicated that medicine helped her maintain her weight. March 24, 1999, it was observed, "I think her spasticity is being helped with the cannabis." April 23, 1999, she continued to get good relief with 10 cigarettes a day. June 24, 1999, the patient reported some increasing difficulty with walking in the heat and hot weather. July 20, 1999, she was said to have no tremor or spasticity. September 1, 1999, she was having some exacerbation and difficulty walking and limping because her right leg was not working as well. October 20, 1999, the patient reported the only bad side effect would be when she smoked too much she would tend to go to sleep. She discussed alternative treatments for multiple sclerosis with her doctor and they agreed not to pursue them. November 19, 1999, the patient was walking on a wide base felt to be the result of a mild exacerbation. November 24, 1999 neurological examination confirmed greater ataxia. Methylphenidate was prescribed. December 1, 1999, an MRI of the brain was said to reveal multiple focal white matter changes in bilateral cerebral areas especially in the basal ganglia and in the cerebellar peduncle, compatible with MS. January 12, 2000, the patient was tried on Ritalin® (methylphenidate). She was switched to Remeron® (mirtazapine) from fluoxetine. February 22, 2000, the patient reported that her eyes were improved. March 9, 2000, visual acuity was 20/200 OD and 20/80 OS. April 6, 2000, it was felt that she had no declines in function from cannabis use. June 27, 2000, her cannabis had been late coming in and she had cut from 10 to 6 or 7 cigarettes a day, feeling that that had hurt her physically and that she was not walking as well. January 31, 2001, the patient was a little bit down and labile, but by February 28, 2001, she was not depressed or hyper. April 11, 2001, she was having some trouble walking due to a flare of symptoms, which had been present for a month, but she noted no changes in vision.

When the patient was interviewed by EBR (June 2001), she reported that her vision was currently clear with cannabis. She was able to ambulate without aids, but has to stop after a block or less due to weakness. She swims a few days a week. She feels that there is no nystagmus in her vision and no diplopia. She characterizes her MS as mildly progressive.

The patient indicated that she received the cannabis legally in 1991 and continues to smoke 10 cigarettes a day. She currently receives material of 3.5% THC content that was processed April 1999. Her study physician requests the highest potency material available, which has recently varied between 2.9-3.7% THC. When she uses outside cannabis of higher potency, she feels that she gets twice the relaxation. There is no chronic cough or other difficulties. The patient feels that Marinol® at 10 mg was too strong. She used it for 6 months before the cannabis. Customarily she splits each of her supplied cigarettes in two, and manicures it slightly. When she is not on cannabis she has had no withdrawal symptoms, but has had increase in movement problems. The patient has had a tubal ligation. She continues to menstruate on a regular monthly basis.

Her main problems have been depression and some degree of anxiety. I asked about other diagnoses and she replied that she had "10 personalities and they are all feeling fine!" She denied history of diabetes, thyroid problems, meningitis, encephalitis, head trauma or seizures. The patient remains on fluoxetine 40 mg a day. She is allergic to penicillin. The patient had 1 year of college. She is right handed.

Family history is noteworthy for father having narcolepsy and a sister who is bipolar.

Social History: She had one child by choice. The patient is a retired clothier, and is unable to work at this time. She is currently smoking ½ pack of cigarettes a day, previously 1 pack a day, and has smoked since age 20. The patient does not drink at all, has not for 5 years, nor has she ever had a problem with alcohol. She does not drink coffee. She customarily sleeps 8 hours.

Medical Test Results: The patient is 5 feet tall and 97 pounds (BMI: 19). On pulmonary function tests, an FVC was 79% of predicted, and FEV 1 76% of predicted. The FEV 1 /FVC was 86. There was felt to be no obstruction based on this ratio or analysis of the F/V curve morphology. Early small airway disease and borderline restrictive disease (e.g., due to MS) were not excluded.

A CBC was wholly within normal limits. An absolute lymphocyte count was 2.3 with CD4 of 58% and CD4 absolute count of 1325. An endocrine battery was performed, with values of FSH, LH, prolactin, estradiol, estrone, estrogen, testosterone and progesterone, all within normal limits for age and gender (pre-menopausal female).

Neuropsychological tests were performed in her home on June 17, 2001. Some confusion was noted throughout the evaluation and significant fatigue over the course of the day was also apparent. She did not have significant difficulty with instructions, however, and effort and cooperation were sufficient to obtain what is believed to be valid data.

As a result of significant visual deficits, many visually based tests were omitted and interpretations from those requiring significant visual input were provided in a very cautious manner. For example, this patient required a magnifying glass in order to accomplish the Picture Completion and Trails subtests that very likely had a significant negative impact on her overall performance.

On the WAIS-III, the patient obtained a Verbal IQ of 93. A Performance IQ was not calculated secondary to significant visual deficits that interfered with assessment in this realm. On the WMS-III, the patient performed, on verbal measures, in the Low Average Range. Immediate auditory memory was at the 18th percentile, with an auditory delayed index in the Average Range. Her ability to acquire non-thematically-organized verbal material was in the mildly impaired range relative to age-matched peers, but her retention was actually very good. Also, she did very well on a test measuring her ability to acquire verbal paired associates with a learning slope actually in the above average range, and excellent retention. Her ability to acquire more detailed and non-thematically-organized verbal information was moderately-to-severely impaired relative to age-matched peers. Overall performances on the CVLT ranged from two to five standard deviations below expected levels. Numerous intrusions during both free and cued recall were noted at levels above and beyond what is generally seen in the normative population.

She made eight false-positive errors on recognition testing, which are also an abnormally high number of errors. Concentration was noted to be markedly impaired in this patient, following the mildly-to-moderately impaired range overall. Assessment of Executive Functions reveals that abstract concept formation and logical analysis abilities were significantly reduced, falling in the moderately impaired range overall. The patient was also noted to be quite perseverative, having difficulty shifting cognitive strategies. In slight contrast, flexibility of thought as measured by the Similarities Subtest from the WAIS-III, was within normal limits. Verbal Fluency was within normal limits relative to age and education-matched peers.

In summary, this patient appears to have decrements in concentration, low average learning, and memory efficiency for new thematic material and verbal paired associates. Her ability to acquire more detailed and non-thematically-organized verbal information is at least moderately impaired. Memory functions, however, appear to be normal in the sense that once she acquires information, she seems to hold it quite effectively. Higher-level executive functions are reduced at a moderate level despite a very remarkable psychiatric history. Responses to the BDI-II were well within normal limits. Patient D thus demonstrates numerous neurocognitive impairments. The general pattern is not particularly uncommon in the context of multiple sclerosis and significant psychiatric dysfunction. This profile, when combined with the others from the data set do not provide any consistent pattern that one could reasonably ascribe to the therapeutic use of cannabis.

Review of Neuropsychological and Cognitive Data
The scientific study of the effects of chronic cannabis on cognition has remained problematical since such concerns were first raised. Despite intensive effort in this regard, little in the way of "hard findings" or consistent results has emerged. A complete review of alleged problems is beyond the scope of this article, but a few citations are meritorious.

In the Jamaican studies (Rubin and Comitas, 1975), 19 neuropsychological tests were administered to chronic cannabis users and controls with no major significant differences between groups. In fact, ganja smokers scored the highest on Wechsler Adult Intelligence Scale (WAIS) Digit Span performance ($p < 0.05$). The authors concluded (p. 119), "in a wide variety of human abilities, there is no evidence that long-term use of cannabis is related to chronic impairment."

In Greece (Kokkevi and Dornbush, 1977), no differences were noted between hashish users and age and socio-economically matched controls in total or Performance IQ (PIQ) scores on the WAIS. Controls performed better on three subtests: Comprehension ($p < 0.01$), Similarities ($p < 0.005$), and Digit Symbol Substitution ($p < 0.05$). Control Verbal IQ (VIQ) surpassed that of users ($p < 0.05$). However, these results must be viewed in light of the fact that normal population studies in Greece revealed PIQ:VIQ differences of 7 points. Thus, the authors concluded, "These observations do not provide evidence of deterioration of mental abilities in the hashish users."

In Costa Rica, an extensive battery of neuropsychological measures showed no pathological changes (Carter, 1980). It was observed, "we failed to uncover significant differences between user and nonuser groups—even in those subjects who had consumed cannabis for over eighteen years."

Subsequently follow-up studies were performed on some of this cohort, and certain significant differences were claimed, including learning of word lists and selective and divided attention tasks (Fletcher, et al., 1996). However, a detailed critical analysis of those results in *Marijuana Myths, Marijuana Facts* (Zimmer and Morgan, 1997) seems to deflate any such claim.

Lyketsos et al. (1999) studied effects of cannabis on cognition in 1318 adults over a period of 12 years. No differences were noted in the degree of decline between heavy, light, and non-users of cannabis on the Mini-Mental State Examination (MMSE). Critics have indicated that the latter represents too crude a tool to measure the issue properly.

In a series of studies in the 1990's summarized in a book, *Cannabis and Cognitive Functioning* (Solowij, 1998), Nadia Solowij studied subjects employing cannabis at least twice a week on average for a period of 3 years. After a review of data, the author stated, "the weight of the evidence suggests that the long-term use of cannabis does not result in any severe or grossly debilitating impairment of cognitive function." She did note more subtle difficulties in attention parameters including distraction, loose associations and intrusion errors in memory tasks. In a recent review of cognitive effects of cannabis (Solowij and Grenyer, 2001), it was observed, "the long term risks for most users are not severe and their effects are relatively subtle...."

Results from the current study seem to indicate similar findings. As part of a Comprehensive Neuropsychological Evaluation, all subjects were administered a battery of instruments including the WAIS-III, the WMS-III, the CVLT, the Trail Making Test A and B, Grooved Peg Board, Finger Tapping, and Category Test, the Controlled Oral Word Association Test, the Thurstone Word Fluency Test, a Category Fluency Test (Animal Naming), the WCST, the CPT-II, and the Beck Depression Inventory–2nd Edition (BDI-II).

Comparing Patients A-D, it appears that all four do have at least mild difficulty with attention and concentration, and verbal acquisition of varying complex new verbal material (as measured on the CVLT), which is at least minimally impaired. Importantly, however, higher-level executive functions generally appear to be within normal limits in two of the subjects.

Difficulties in attention and concentration as well as new complex verbal learning may be directly related, and must be understood in the context of not only these subjects' chronic cannabis use, but also their underlying chronic diseases and clinical syndromes, with attendant fatigue and preoccupation. Interestingly, depressive symptoms are not currently noted at a clinical level in any of the subjects despite their chronic medical conditions or long-term cannabis use. None displayed evidence of social withdrawal or apathy characteristic of the alleged "amotivational syndrome." Rather, all were animated, engaging in conversation and demonstrating an active involvement with their ongoing care and the current research.

Overall, once more, no significant attributable neuropsychological sequelae are noted due to chronic cannabis usage.

Review of Neuroimaging
In 1971, it was reported that "consistent cannabis smoking" of 3-11 years in ten patients produced evidence for cerebral atrophy employing air encephalography (Campbell, et al., 1971), an excruciatingly painful and long abandoned technique. A subsequent study employing CT scans on 19 men with long durations of heavy cannabis usage failed to show any changes in the ventricles or sub-arachnoid spaces (Kuehnle, et al., 1977). Kuehnle criticized the prior study for lacking controls on antecedent head trauma or other causes of neurological damage. In the same issue of the *Journal of the American Medical Association*, another study revealed an additional 12 heavy cannabis smokers who displayed no CT abnormalities (Co, et al., 1977).

In 1983, an additional 12 subjects who smoked more than 1 g of cannabis daily for 10 years were studied by CT scans of the brain, and only one with concomitant history of alcoholism showed any abnormalities compared to controls (Hannerz and Hindmarsh, 1983).

Most recently, Block et al. (2000) employed automated imaging analysis with MRI to examine 18 young heavy users of cannabis. No abnormalities were ascertained. The authors stated, "Frequent marijuana use does not produce clinically apparent MRI abnormalities or detectable global or regional changes in brain tissue volumes of gray or white matter, or both combined." It was recently noted (Solowij and Grenyer, 2001, p. 270), "There is no evidence from human studies of any structural brain damage following prolonged exposure to cannabinoids."

Despite this additional documentation, the claim of brain damage and cerebral atrophy remains a popular myth in prohibitionist rhetoric.

Current MRI studies on Patients A-C with a General Electric Sigma LX MR 1.5 Tesla magnet system reveal no clear abnormalities. Patient A had age-compatible atrophy, and Patient C had minor tissue changes of a non-specific nature, commonly seen in middle-aged populations. Patient D has previously demonstrated

MRI brain lesions consistent with MS, with possible improvement observed during the period of clinical cannabis usage.

Review of Neurophysiology Tests

In discussing the issue of cannabis and cerebral effects, Homer Reed observed (Reed, 1975, pp. 122-123), "The association between many of the EEG measures used to indicate CNS changes and the clinical condition of the patient is approximately zero." That not withstanding, various researchers have advanced numerous claims of pertinent EEG changes due to cannabis. Cohen (1976) noted differences in computerized EEG measures of delta band power and theta band phase angle (lead/lag) relationship. No mention was made of the alleged significance of these tests, or of the results of standard EEG.

All the Jamaican subjects had EEG examinations (Rubin and Comitas, 1975). As previously noted in other studies, 9 of 30 cannabis smokers had significant low voltage fast activity in the beta range. Although this finding may indicate sedative effects of medication, it is often ascribed to a normal variant. Three of the 30 were said to have unequivocal focal abnormalities, but 4 of 30 controls had similar findings, and another had diffuse abnormalities. Overall, no significant differences were noted between ganja smokers and controls.

Similarly, in Greece (Panayiotopoulos, et al., 1977), 8.8% of 46 hashish smokers had abnormal EEGs, while 15% of 40 normal controls were so characterized. The authors stated, "We failed to find either an abnormality or an particular EEG change in the resting EEG records of chronic hashish users...."

Current results, performed on a 21-channel Nicolet Voyageur digital EEG system and read by EBR, confirm the presence of low voltage fast activity in Patients A-C, and intermittent sharp waves and rare subtle slowing in the left frontal area in Patient A. Age appropriate atrophy was seen in the same patient on MRI, but she has no history of seizures or CNS insults. There are no corresponding abnormalities on neurological examination. Similar abnormalities are identified on EEGs of 6% of patients, whereas there is only a 0.5% prevalence of seizure disorders in the general population. In essence, no EEG pathology of an attributable nature seems apparent in the study group on the basis of cannabis usage.

With respect to P300 responses, a type of electrophysiological event related potential, even greater caution is necessary. This parameter is offered as an electrophysiological measure of memory, inasmuch as prolongation of its latency occurs with age. The test was popular in the 1980s as an objective test for dementia. Amplitude differences have also been noted in different clinical conditions, but were termed (Spehlmann, 1985, p. 370), "of uncertain diagnostic importance because of the great normal variability of the P300 amplitude." Overall, these issues and significant incidence of false positives and false negatives have largely relegated use of this technique to the sidelines as a clinical tool.

Solowij (1998) studied the P300 in chronic cannabis users vs. controls, and noted results felt to be indicative of, "inefficient processing of information and impaired selective attention." These consisted of reduced processing negativity to relevant attended stimuli, inappropriately large processing negativity to a source of complex irrelevant stimuli, and reduced P300 amplitude to attended target stimuli to that of controls.

In contrast, Patrick, et al. (1995) examined the P300 in psychologically normal chronic cannabis users and controlled the data for age. Results showed no amplitude differences.

More recent studies have shown significant reductions in P300 amplitude in schizophrenia (Martin-Loeches, et al., 2001), but also in cigarette smokers (Anokhin, et al., 2000), with notable effects according to motivational instructions (Carrillo-de-la-Pena and Cadaveira, 2000), and even diurnal variations (Higuchi, et al., 2000).

Our study employed a Nicolet Viking 3P 4-channel system with a P300 oddball paradigm. Patients A-C displayed P300 latencies that were well within norms for age-matched controls.

Review of Pulmonary Issues

Pulmonary concerns remain paramount in relation to chronic cannabis smoking. Excellent recent reviews are available (Zimmer and Morgan, 1997; Tashkin, 2001; Tashkin, 2001). In brief, cannabis smoking produces an increase in cough and bronchitis symptoms, but to a lesser degree than in tobacco smokers (Sherrill, et al., 1991). Daily cannabis smokers seek medical care for smoking-associated health concerns at a slightly higher rate than non-smokers (Polen, et al., 1993). In a large epidemiological study, cannabis use was associated with little statistical association on total mortality in women, and non-AIDS mortality in men (Sidney, et al., 1997).

One of the primary associated risks of tobacco smoking is the development of emphysema and lesser declines in bronchial function over time. A careful longitudinal study of chronic smokers has demonstrated a longitudinal decline in the FEV 1 in tobacco smokers, but not heavy cannabis smokers (Tashkin, et al., 1997).

Some association of cannabis smoking has been observed to head and neck cancers (Zhang, et al., 1999), and pre-cancerous cytological changes have been noted in the lungs in bronchoscopy studies (Fligiel, et al., 1988), but to date, no cases of pulmonary carcinoma have been noted in cannabis-only smokers.

In examining the data from chronic cannabis use studies, in Jamaica, a slight downward trend not attaining statistical significance was noted on forced vital capacity (FVC) values (Rubin and Comitas, 1975). A similar downward trend was observed on FEV 1 without statistical significance.

No differences between cannabis smokers, occasional smokers and non-smokers were observed on FEV 1/FVC ratios. Results of all tests may have been affected by concomitant tobacco usage.

The Greek studies did not closely examine pulmonary function, and although an increase in bronchitis symptoms was noted in hashish smokers over abstainers, the former group also smoked more tobacco. Differences were not statistically significant in any event (Boulougouris, Antypas and Panayiotopoulos, 1977).

In the Costa Rican studies, no spirometry measures were significantly different between cannabis users and non-users. However, statistical trends were, in fact, positive with respect to cannabis usage. Cannabis smokers displayed larger indices of small-airway patency. The authors suggested that in concomitant smoking of tobacco, cannabis seemed to counteract the expected effects of tobacco on small air-ways. The author stated (Carter, 1980, p. 171), "at least it cannot be said of the users that they have suffered an additive of [sic-"or"] synergistic decrement in pulmonary function over that attributable to tobacco alone."

In our Patients A-C, no ultimate chest radiographic changes of significance were noted, despite a false-positive reading of pulmonary nodule in Patient C. It is of particular note that he has had a previous bronchoscopy procedure with no reported cytological changes.

Observed pulmonary function values in this cohort reveal no clear trends except a slight downward trend in FEV 1 and FEV 1/FVC ratios, and perhaps an increase in FVC (Patients A-C) (Table 3). Concomitant tobacco smoking (Patients A, B and D) complicates analysis. It is particularly interesting that Patient B, a current concomitant smoker of tobacco displayed the best spirometry values, while those in Patient C, a never-smoker of tobacco were the worst. His underlying connective tissue disease may have played an active role in this finding. His use of the lowest grade cannabis and highest amount per day are the more likely explanation.

Significant questions remain as to the role of low-grade NIDA cannabis as a contributor to the above findings, which will subsequently discussed.

Review of Hematological Studies
No effects on complete blood counts or hemoglobin were observed in the LaGuardia Commission report (New York, NY). Mayor's committee on mari-

huana (Wallace and Cunningham, 1944). In the Jamaican studies, slight increases were observed in hematocrit and hemoglobin readings in cannabis smokers over controls, but results were affected by concomitant tobacco use (Rubin and Comitas, 1975). No hematological data was obtained from the Greek studies. In Costa Rica, a downward trend was observed in hematocrit readings of cannabis smokers, but this was not statistically noteworthy (Carter, 1980).

In our studies (Table 4), Patient B, a concomitant tobacco smoker, displayed a mild degree of polycythemia and slightly elevated WBC. No other hematological changes of any type were evident in the other three patients.

Review of Immunological Parameters

Immune system damage remains an area of contention with respect to cannabis usage (Zimmer and Morgan, 1997), but one in which there is considerably more heat than light. A closer examination of the available literature may allay concern. In the chronic use studies in Jamaica, no decrement was observed in cannabis smokers vs. controls in either lymphocyte or neutrophils counts (Rubin and Comitas, 1975). Neither were significant changes noted in the data in Costa Rica (Carter, 1980).

In the 94-Day Cannabis Study, initial acute low values were observed in T cell counts, but these returned to normal over the course of the testing (Cohen 1976). A closer examination of the pertinent literature raises concerns on theoretical levels to a greater degree than practical ones. Excellent reviews are available (Klein, Friedman, and Specter, 1998; Hollister, 1992; Cabral, 2001; Cabral, 2001).

Early reports of inhibition of cell mediated immunity in cannabis smokers (Nahas, et al., 1974) were refuted by later studies in which no impairment of lymphocytic response to phytohemagglutinin in hashish smokers was observed (Kaklamani, et al., 1978).

A seminal review of the topic was undertaken by Hollister (1992), who stated (p. 159), "Evidence of altered immune functions is derived mainly from in vitro tests or ex vivo experiments, which employed doses of cannabinoids far in excess of those that prevail during social use of marijuana." More recently, Klein, Friedman and Specter (1998) have similarly noted, "Although cannabinoids modulate immune cell function, it is also clear that these cells are relatively resistant to the drugs in that many effects appear to be relatively small and totally reversible, occur at concentration higher than needed to induce psychoactivity (>10 μM or >5 mg/kg), and occur following treatment with nonpsychoactive cannabinoid analogues." They added, "The public health risk of smoking marijuana in terms of increased susceptibility to infections, especially opportunistic infections, is still unclear."

Finally, despite concerns raised by THC effects on immunity in animals and *in vitro*, Cabral and Dove Pettit (1998) admitted (p. 116), "Definitive data which directly link marijuana use to increased susceptibility to infection in humans cur-rently is unavailable."

A particular public health concern surrounds cannabis effects on HIV/AIDS. Four studies among others may reduce related concern.

Kaslow, et al. (1989) demonstrated no evidence that cannabis accelerated immun-odeficiency parameters in HIV-positive patients. Di Franco, et al. (1996) ascer-tained no acceleration of HIV to full-blown AIDS in cannabis smokers. Whitfield, Bechtel and Starich (1997) observed no deleterious effects of cannabis usage in HIV/AIDS patients, even those with the lowest CD4 counts. Finally, Abrams et al. (2000) studied the effects of cannabis smoking on HIV positive patients on protease inhibitor drugs in a prospective randomized, partially blinded placebo controlled trial. No adverse effects on CD4 counts were observed secondary to cannabis.

In our studies of four subjects (Table 4), Patient B had an elevated WBC count, prob-ably attributable to the stress of phlebotomy, but without accompanying disorders of cell count differential. All patients had CD4 counts well within normal limits.

Review of Endocrine Function

Topical reviews of this topic are contained in two recent publications (Murphy, 2001; Zimmer and Morgan, 1997). As with other physiological systems, much data is based on animal studies, and early claims of deleterious effects on acute endocrine function are not necessarily supported by subsequent investigations or chronic use studies.

One long held claim is the production of gynecomastia in males associated with cannabis use. A case study of 3 cannabis smokers with this malady was reported by Harmon and Aliapoulios (1972). A more thorough investigation a few years later failed to show any differences in cannabis use in affected males between users and controls (Cates and Pope 1977). Similarly, Kolodny, et al. (1974) reported decreased testosterone levels in chronic marijuana smokers, while no differences in testosterone or luteinizing hormone (LH) levels were identified in a 3-week trial of smokers vs. non-smokers (Mendelson, et al., 1978). LH levels in menopausal women showed no significant changes after cannabis usage (Mendelson, et al., 1985), but the next year, a similar group noted a 30% sup-pression of LH in women by smoking a single cannabis cigarette during the luteal phase (Mendelson, et al., 1986). Subsequently, a more in-depth study of both sexes was undertaken to assess multiple hormone effects comparing subjects with different levels of cannabis usage vs. controls (Block, Farinpour, and Schlechte

1991). No significant effects were noted on testosterone, LH, FSH, prolactin or cortisol in young women and men.

Jamaican chronic use studies were confined to examinations of thyroxine and steroid excretion with no significant findings observed due to cannabis use (Rubin and Comitas, 1975).

In the 94-Day Cannabis Study, acute drops in testosterone and LH levels were noted after smoking a cannabis cigarette (Cohen, 1976). Subsequent drops in testosterone levels were noted after the 5th week of daily usage. LH levels fell after the 4th week and FSH after the 8th week to unspecified degrees.

In Costa Rica, no differences were noted in male testosterone levels between abstainers and cannabis smokers stratified according to amount of use (Carter, 1980). Similarly, fertility was unimpaired, with both groups having identical numbers of progeny. The author stated (p. 172), "These findings cast serious doubt on cause-and-effect relationship between marihuana smoking and plasma testosterone level in long-term use." Zimmer and Morgan (1997) summarized their observations by stating (p. 92), "There is no scientific evidence that marijuana delays adolescent sexual development, has a feminizing effect on males, or a masculinizing effect on females."

The latter statement would seem to be borne out by our findings. While one male subject had a minor degree of gynecomastia associated with obesity, none of the Patients A-D displayed any abnormal values in any endocrine measure. Patient A has two children, Patient B has three, and Patient D had one by choice.

Problems in the Compassionate IND Program

All four patients described varying degrees of logistical difficulties in obtaining their medicine. All have to travel or make special arrangements with their study physician, who is the arbiter of the potency of received material. All described incidents of inadequate supply or provision of inferior quality cannabis. All have had to supplement their supplies of cannabis from illegal black market sources at times. All have experienced inconveniences or security concerns when traveling. One, Patient C, was arrested, detained, and had some of his medicine permanently confiscated without replacement. Patients A-C decried the lack of an official identity card that might be readily recognized and accepted by law enforcement and security personnel. Rather, all used combinations of letters and other documents to convey their legal status to interested authorities, often to the accompaniment of much doubt and suspicion. All describe significant worry and anxiety about their medicine supplies, and whether official promises of continuation of the program will be honored.

A paramount issue affecting the Compassionate IND patients revolves around cannabis quality. It has been well established that recreational cannabis smokers prefer higher potency materials (Herning, Hooker, and Jones, 1986; Chait and Burke, 1994; Kelly, et al. 1997). The same pertains for most clinical cannabis patients. Chait and Pierri (1989) published a detailed analysis of NIDA marijuana cigarettes that is worthy of review in this context. NIDA marijuana is grown outside, one crop per biennium, harvested from a 5-acre facility at the University of Mississippi. Average yield of "manicured material" is 270 g per plant or 270 g per square foot (letter from NIDA, Steven Gust to Chris Conrad, August 18, 1999). Material is shipped to the Research Triangle Institute in North Carolina where it is chopped and rolled on modified tobacco cigarette machines, then stored partially dehydrated and frozen. Cigarettes average 800-900 g in weight. Material requires rehydration before usage, which the IND patients usually achieve by storage overnight in a refrigerated plastic bag with leaves of lettuce.

As of 1999 (letter, Steven Gust to EBR, June 7, 1999), NIDA had available cannabis cigarettes of 1.8%, 2.8%, 3.0%, and 3.4% THC, and bulk cannabis of up to 5% THC content. Other cannabinoid components were not quantitated. It was further stated that the strongest material was not provided to patients in their cigarette shipments because it was too sticky and would interfere with the rolling machine's functioning (Personal Communication to EBR, Steven Gust, December 1999).

Static burn rates of NIDA cannabis cigarettes were inversely related to potency (Chait and Pierri, 1989), while the number of puffs that could be drawn from each cigarette averaged 8.8. While total particulate matter increased with potency, arguably less smoked material is necessary for medicinal effect. Of more concern, carbon monoxide levels were highest in the lower potency material; that is, CO was inversely proportional to THC content. Finally, test subjects in their study of NIDA cannabis reported (pp. 66-67), "that the marijuana is inferior in sensory qualities (taste, harshness) than the marijuana that they smoke outside the laboratory. Some have stated that it was the worst marijuana they had ever sampled, or that it tasted 'chemically treated.' "

All the study patients criticize the paper employed to roll the cannabis cigarettes as harsh, and tasting poorly. NIDA cannabis cigarettes resemble Pall Mall® brand tobacco cigarettes without the logo. All study patients clean their cannabis and re-roll the material to varying degrees, although at least one former IND patient, now deceased, used the NIDA cigarettes unaltered.

NIDA cannabis is shipped to patients in labeled metal canisters containing 300 cigarettes, and material is frequently two or more years old upon receipt. Even under optimal storage conditions, a certain degree of oxidation of cannabinoids can be expected (Grotenhermen, 2001). Most consumers prefer a supply of cured cannabis that is as fresh as possible.

A close inspection of the contents of NIDA-supplied cannabis cigarettes reveals them to be a crude mixture of leaf with abundant stem and seed components. The odor is green and herbal in character. The resultant smoke is thick, acrid, and pervasive. In contrast, a typical sinsemilla "bud" is seedless, covered with visible glandular trichomes, and emits a strong lemony or piney terpenoid scent. The smoke is also less disturbing from a sensory standpoint to most observers.

Whittle, Guy, and Robson (2001) describe in detail the markedly contrasting steps undertaken in a government approved clinical cannabis program in the United Kingdom. Their material is organically grown in soil with no chemical treatment under controlled indoor conditions. All male plants are eliminated, and only unfertilized female flowering tops are harvested for further processing. This material is assayed for cannabinoid and terpenoid content, with controlled ratios through genetic selection of seed strains before extraction. THC yields obtained are routinely 15-20% (Personal Communication, GW Pharmaceuticals, 2000).

Harm reduction techniques in relation to clinical cannabis consumption are well advanced (Russo 2001; Grotenhermen, 2001a, 2001b). Particular attention is merited toward vaporization techniques that provide cannabinoid and terpenoid component administration to prospective clinical cannabis patients without pyrolysis (Gieringer, 1996a; Gieringer, 1996b; Gieringer, 2001). Sublingual administration of cannabis extracts is another most promising technique of clinical cannabis administration (Whittle, Guy, and Robson, 2001).

Three of the four study subjects have employed Marinol®, and found it inadequate or a poor substitute for cannabis in symptomatic relief of their clinical syndromes.

CONCLUSIONS AND RECOMMENDATIONS

1. Cannabis smoking, even of a crude, low-grade product, provides effective symptomatic relief of pain, muscle spasms, and intra-ocular pressure elevations in selected patients failing other modes of treatment.

2. These clinical cannabis patients are able to reduce or eliminate other prescription medicines and their accompanying side effects.

3. Clinical cannabis provides an improved quality of life in these patients.

4. The side effect profile of NIDA cannabis in chronic usage suggests some mild pulmonary risk.

5. No malignant deterioration has been observed.

6. No consistent or attributable neuropsychological or neurological deterioration has been observed.

7. No endocrine, hematological or immunological sequelae have been observed.

8. Improvements in a clinical cannabis program would include a ready and consistent supply of sterilized, potent, organically grown, unfertilized, female flowering top material, thoroughly cleaned of extraneous inert fibrous matter.

9. It is the authors' opinion that the Compassionate IND program should be reopened and extended to other patients in need of clinical cannabis.

10. Failing that, local, state and federal laws might be amended to provide regulated and monitored clinical cannabis to suitable candidates.

REFERENCES
Abrams, D., R. Leiser, T. Mitchell, J. Aberg, S. Deeks, and S. Shade. 2000. Short-term effects of cannabinoids in human immunodeficiency virus (HIV) infection: Clinical safety results. Paper read at 2000 Symposium on the Cannabinoids, June 23, 2000, at Hunt Valley, MD.

B
Appendix

Condensed Excerpt from Supreme Court Transcripts of Oral Arguments in United States vs. Oakland Cannabis Buyers' Cooperative

Question: I gather cannabis is not a life-saving drug. It alleviates great pain and discomfort.

Mr. Uelmen: Well, we believe it is a life-saving drug. It's a life-saving drug for AIDS patients who are not going to benefit from the new medications available to keep them alive if they can't keep their weight up, if they can't maintain their general health.

Question: So how serious—how serious does a case have to be before this medical-necessity defense kicks in, in your view?

Mr. Uelmen: Well, in the injunction we're talking in terms of imminent harm, we believe that—

Question: What sort of harm?

Mr. Uelmen: Death, starvation, blindness.

Question: Stomachache?

Mr. Uelmen: No.

Question: That's a harm, isn't it?

Mr. Uelmen: We're talking about patients who are going to lose their sight, who are going to forego chemotherapy or radiation, because they can't live with the severe nausea.

Question: You have to add some adjective to just imminent harm, you want immanent life-threatening harm, imminent what? You want to exclude a stomachache and an earache, maybe.

Mr. Uelmen: No, I think we're talking about much more serious harm, but we're talking about balancing the choice of evils here...the person who provides the substance to the patient is also faced with a choice of evils.

Question: Well, what choice of evils is the provider faced with?

Mr. Uelmen: Of letting someone die or violating the law.

Question: Well, of not being able to supply the person. I mean it certainly isn't the provider's responsibility to look after the individual.

Mr. Uelmen: Well—

Question: You say letting someone die.

Mr. Uelmen: We're saying the necessity defense permits or justifies this choice even by the provider as well as the patient...a druggist may dispense a drug without the requisite prescription to alleviate grave distress in an emergency...I might point out that it's a business in which the government itself has been engaged. The government provides cannabis at the present time to eight patients who meet essentially the criteria of medical necessity, and—

Question: It's one thing to say that a state law requiring a prescription for a bunch of drugs can be violated in an emergency. It's another thing to say that a schedule one law which says there's no useful medical purpose for this drug shall be violated.

Mr. Uelmen: Well, the government's position actually is that there is no necessity defense for any drug under the Controlled Substances Act, and I think it is very important that the court realize that the reason why we're here is because the government shut down the only program that could accommodate these patients. For many years they provided cannabis and still do for eight patients who come within this medical necessity criteria, and they closed that program down in 1992 and they say in their brief, "we can do it because we're the federal government. You can't do it because you're a private citizen".

Well, we're saying if you won't do it, we can do it because the only justification you have to do it is the same medical necessity defense that we're asserting and the way the necessity defense works is if a patient comes in and says I have to have this to live and the court says, "Well, the government has a program. They'll give it to you. Therefore you have a reasonable alternative." A patient with glaucoma comes into court, asserts a necessity defense. The court says, "You have a reasonable alternative," and that patient then goes to the government and they put him on the Compassionate IND program and provide him with cannabis. Well, now the government decides we're not going to operate this program anymore, and we say if you're not going to do it then we can, because the only justification you had to do it was this medical necessity defense concept.

There is no authorization within the Controlled Substances Act for the government to give cannabis as medicine to patients...I especially invite the Court to carefully look at the hearings held by Congress on the therapeutic uses of marijuana...

‖ C

Appendix

Provision of Marijuana and Other Compounds For Scientific Research Recommendations of The National Institute on Drug Abuse National Advisory Council

January, 1998

ISSUE: Since its inception in 1974, NIDA has been the sole administrator of a contract to grow cannabis (marijuana) for research purposes and the only legal source for cannabis in the United States. Scientific studies require a source of cannabis materials that have consistent and predictable potency, are free of contamination, and are available in amounts to support research needs. During the 1970s the demand for cannabis materials was high. As much became known from science about the pharmacology of cannabis and its biomedical and behavioral effects, less cannabis research was done and demand for cannabis materials declined markedly. In the last decade or so the research demand has remained relatively low, such that available supply has exceeded the demand. However, recent State initiatives and an NIH-wide scientific workshop in February 1997 co-sponsored by ten NIH components have generated increased interest in research related to the potential medical uses of cannabis. Thus, there may soon be an increase in requests. Some of these requests will come from NIDA grantees or grantees of other NIH Institutes, which guarantees both a peer and Council review. Others, however, may come from individuals receiving State or private funding and may not have undergone equivalent scientific peer review. As a result of these recent developments, it has become important for NIDA to reevaluate its policies related to the Drug Supply Program, and in particular the growing and supplying of cannabis, to ensure that reviews of all proposals are objective, uniform, rigorous, and appropriate, and are so viewed by the disparate communities of interest. Accordingly, there is a need for Council to develop a set of procedures and guidelines on practical and policy issues related to the provision of cannabis.

BACKGROUND: In 1968, the National Institute of Mental Health began funding a Drug Supply Program to provide researchers with compounds necessary to conduct biomedical research. Initially, the program focused on THC and other naturally occurring cannabinoids, and then gradually expanded to a wide range of compounds. (Since its beginning, the program has synthesized or obtained over 1,500 different compounds that have been supplied to over 2,500 researchers.) Cannabis was among the first substances to be made available through the Drug Supply Program for use by scientists conducting both nonhuman research and human research under a variety of investigational new drug protocols. It was grown through a contract with the University of Mississippi. With its establishment in 1974, NIDA became the successor to NIMH as the administrator of the cannabis contract and the sole U.S. source for legal cannabis. NIDA has continued to grow cannabis in order to provide a contamination-free source of cannabis material with consistent and predictable potency for use in biomedical research. Because of international treaty agreements (Single Convention on Narcotic Drugs, 1961) which prohibit entities other than the Federal Government from legally supplying cannabis, NIDA has remained its only legal source. These same treaty agreements as well as DEA regulations require that only the amounts of cannabis needed for medical and research purposes be produced. In addition to the contract with the University of Mississippi, NIDA also supports two contracts with the Research Triangle Institute (RTI) for, among other purposes, the manufacture and distribution of standardized cannabis cigarettes.

NIDA also supplies cannabis to seven patients under single patient so-called "compassionate use" Investigational New Drug Applications (IND). In 1978, as part of a lawsuit settlement by the Department of Health and Human Services, NIDA began supplying cannabis to patients whose physicians applied for and received such an USID from the FDA. In 1992, the Secretary terminated this practice, but decided that NIDA should continue to supply those patients who were receiving cannabis at the time.

Under the current contract with the University of Mississippi for any given year NIDA has the option to grow either 1.5 or 6.5 acres of cannabis, or to not grow any at all, depending on research demand. Generally, 1.5 acres are grown in alternate years. The number of cannabis cigarettes produced from 1.5 acres is about 50,000-60,000, although it can be higher. Cigarettes are produced in three potencies: strength 1 - 3-4 %; strength 2 - 1.8-2.2 %; and strength 3 - placebo, as close to 0% as possible. During the past three years, the following quantities have been shipped: 1994 - 24,000 cigarettes; 1995 - 23,100 - cigarettes; and 1996 17,700 cigarettes. Virtually all of the cigarettes shipped in the last three years have been for single patient INDs. As of March 1997 there were 278,100 cigarettes in stock. The cigarettes are maintained in frozen storage and have a useful life of approximately five years.

The contract with the University of Mississippi funds the growing, harvesting and storage of cannabis. It also funds potency monitoring and other services for the DEA. The total contract, including DEA activities, is about $480,000 during growing years and $350,000 during nongrowing years. Of these amounts the costs associated with cannabis are about $362,000 during growing years (for 1.5 acres) and $232,000 during nongrowing years. The remaining $118,000/year (approximately) of the contract is used for DEA activities and is not associated with the growing of cannabis.

There are currently two contracts with RTI. One of these, totaling $615,571/year, funds the manufacture of cannabis cigarettes, as well as the analysis of cannabis material, and the development and production of standardized reconstituted cannabinoid preparations. About 10% of this contract ($61,557/year) is for the manufacture of cannabis cigarettes.

These costs from the contracts with the University of Mississippi and RTI that are associated with the growing of cannabis and the production and shipping of cigarettes are approximately $420,000 during a growing year and $300,000 during a nongrowing year. Funding at this level allows for the production of cannabis cigarettes with a uniform potency and purity, consistency of seed stock, the analysis of THC content and adjustments when necessary, and other activities crucial to the production of research grade cannabis cigarettes.

If it were necessary, NIDA could exercise a contract option with the University of Mississippi to grow an additional five acres at a cost of $310,000. Additional costs would then also be incurred in the RTI contract for the production of the cannabis cigarettes.

The other RTI contract for $1,735,400/year funds the synthesis and analysis of other compounds that are available through NIDA's Drug Supply Program and the purification of other compounds.

NIDA's present policy is to provide cannabis for medical research purposes to either grantees or nongrantees whose research and protocols have scientific merit, providing the research is determined to be an appropriate use of NIDA resources and the principal investigator obtains the necessary licences. For NIDA-funded projects, the project officer reviews the protocol, determines whether the amounts requested are justified and makes recommendations to the NIDA drug supply officer. If the request is from someone who is not a NIDA grantee, the project is reviewed by two outside experts for scientific merit, protocol, and amount of drug requested. Each reviewer then makes a recommendation as to whether or not NIDA should supply the cannabis. If the outside experts differ in their recommendations, a third expert is asked to review the request. In all cases, if cannabis is supplied, there is no cost to the researcher. NIDA absorbs all of the costs associated with the production and shipping of the cannabis, whether it is being provided to a NIDA grantee or a non-NIDA grantee.

In recent years, growing 1.5 acres every other year has been adequate to supply both the seven patients receiving cannabis under individual patient INDs and cannabis research grants. There are indications now, however, that the number of requests may increase, perhaps dramatically. The Division of Research Grants has already reported the submission of three grant applications that deal directly with studying the medical use of cannabis—one on the short-term effects of cannabinoids in HIV patients, a second on ocular cannabinoid effects, and a third on cannabis in the treatment of acute migraine. In addition, the number of requests from non-NIH applicants also may increase substantially. For example, pursuant to a 1991 law that establishes a Therapeutic Research Program within the Massachusetts State Department of Health and Human Services and a 1996 law that makes it legal for patients in the program to have cannabis in their possession, the Massachusetts Department of Public Health has sought assurances that NIDA will supply cannabis for clinical trials on the plant material as a therapeutic modality. NIDA also has received inquiries from the Executive Director of Special Research Programs at the University of California concerning the provision of cannabis for research purposes. This request is associated with a measure that is currently before the California legislature that would establish a California Medical Cannabis Research Center at the University of California.

An additional consideration relative to the supply of cannabis is the possibility that investigators may request cannabis cigarettes with either a THC potency of greater than 4% or with varying amounts of other cannabinoids. For example, NIDA has received a request for cigarettes with an 8% potency. Currently, the highest potency manufactured is 4%. To obtain the higher potency, NIDA would either have to use more crude material or use special, more costly, growing methods.

CURRENT STATUS: NIDA is evaluating its policies related to the Drug Supply Program, in particular the growing and supplying of cannabis, to ensure consistency and uniformity. The National Advisory Council is being requested to assist NIDA through the development of clear guidelines and policies related to this issue. A subcommittee of the Council has met and determined that the questions listed below should be considered by the full Council. Background and the Council subcommittee recommendations are included for each question.

1.   Who should administer the contracts associated with the growing and production of cannabis?

    BACKGROUND: According to international treaties, only an agency of the Federal government can produce and supply cannabis. Although NIDA has been the responsible Federal agency since 1974, any other Federal agency could assume both the costs and responsibilities of maintaining the farm and supplying cannabis. NIDA's legal authority allows for the provision of cannabis only for drug abuse research purposes. Nonetheless, as a result of the court settlement noted earlier, in addition to providing cannabis for research activities, NIDA also provides cannabis to the seven patients still covered by the single patient INDs.

Over the past few years, there have been very few requests from NIDA grantees for cannabis cigarettes. As a result of expected increases in the number of requests, however, a consideration in who administers the contracts is the dollar cost and its potential impact on the ability to support other NIDA-funded drug abuse research. Further, there now exists a NIDA standard cannabis cigarette that drug abuse researchers can rely on for consistent potency and quality. If NIDA doesn't maintain the farm, there could be less assurance that these standard cannabis cigarettes will continue to be available to NIDA grantees.

COUNCIL SUBCOMMITTEE RECOMMENDATION: The Council subcommittee recommends that NIDA continue to maintain responsibility for the contracts. This would ensure that the quality of the cannabis cigarettes is maintained and that NIDA grantees continue to have a source of cannabis with a uniform consistency.

The subcommittee also recommends that the growing methods be evaluated. The current methods may not be state of the art. Alternative methods, such as hydroponic, may be more efficient. Use of other methods may also make it easier to respond to increases in demand if there is an increase in the number of meritorious requests. The use of newer growing methods would also facilitate the production of varied types and compositions of cannabis cigarettes.

2. What mechanism should be used for determining which researchers should receive cannabis?

BACKGROUND: NIH-funded proposals have been through a rigorous scientific review and have received a priority score based on their merit. NIDA staff can rely on this review to determine whether or not to supply cannabis. Requests from other sources, however, may or may not have been scientifically peer reviewed, and do not have a priority score or indication of feasibility of study design or level of enthusiasm. NIDA policy has been to request two outside evaluations of requests for cannabis that come from outside sources. The reviewers are asked to give a recommendation as to whether or not NIDA should provide cannabis. They do not give the proposal a priority score. It is very likely that the number of requests from non-NIH funded sources will increase markedly and NIDA must be able to clearly justify its decisions. It is therefore important that NIDA evaluate the adequacy of its current review procedures. In doing so, consideration should be given to ensuring that the review procedure is able to handle a large number of requests and to conduct an equivalent review—one as rigorous and comparable to that conducted by an NIH study section as is possible. Attention also must be paid to the process by which scientific experts are selected, such that members of the review panels have scientific expertise related to the disease states being studied, as well clinical pharmacology and therapeutics.

COUNCIL SUBCOMMITTEE RECOMMENDATIONS: The Council subcommittee agrees that NIDA should not have the sole responsibility for determining who should receive cannabis and that other NIH Institutes with an interest in cannabis research should be involved. The subcommittee also recommends that a clear and uniform procedure be established for determining which researchers should received cannabis. It is recommended that this procedure consist of a two stage review. The first stage would involve a review by the funding agency, either NIH or an outside agency or state or local government. Those applications that are determined to be meritorious at the first level of review would then receive a second stage review. This review would focus on the appropriateness of the request for cannabis. Several options are proposed as to how this second stage should be conducted. The preferred mechanism is to establish a standing review committee composed of representatives, from relevant NIH Institutes and outside reviewers. The committee would consist of a core group of scientists that is supplemented, as needed, by ad hoc scientific reviewers with expertise related to specific disease states and/or clinical pharmacology and therapeutics. In order to avoid any delays in funding, this review would take place shortly after IRG review, in the case of NIH grants or shortly after the receipt of the request, in the case on non-NIH grants. The Council subcommittee does not feel it is necessary for grants that are not funded by NIDA to come before the NIDA Council. However, NIDA should provide Council with periodic reports on cannabis requests and usage.

3. Should cannabis continue to be available to researchers at no cost?

BACKGROUND: Presently NIDA absorbs all costs associated with the growth, production and shipping of cannabis, regardless of whether or not the request is from a NIDA-funded investigator. Grants related to research on the medical use of cannabis have already been submitted to other NIH Institutes and a request for cannabis from a non-NIH funded investigator has been submitted to NIDA. If the number of requests continues to increase, the cost to NIDA could be substantial. The use of funds to produce cannabis cigarettes for non-drug abuse research purposes represents a diversion of resources intended for drug abuse research.

NIDA also currently provides services such as potency monitoring and paraquat analysis for the DEA through the cannabis production contracts. In addition, the DEA serves as an intermediary for individuals wishing to acquire cannabis for training dogs to sniff drugs. NIDA receives no compensation for these services.

COUNCIL SUBCOMMITTEE RECOMMENDATION: The subcommittee emphatically agrees that NIDA should not continue to supply cannabis to researchers free of charge. The following are specific recommendations for several types of requestors:

1.   DEA - The subcommittee noted that NIDA's resources are intended to be used for drug abuse related research purposes, but that the DEA activities that are currently funded through NIDA's contract with the University of Mississippi are not research related. The subcommittee therefore recommends that NIDA either receive compensation for DEA activities that are currently funded through the NIDA contracts, or discontinue these activities.

2.   NIH grantees - The subcommittee recommends that NIH grantees reimburse NIDA for the cost of cannabis that they receive. The subcommittee, however, also expresses concern about the impact on indirect costs and ultimately on the cost to the funding Institutes, should cannabis be included in grant costs. It suggests either that cannabis costs be excluded from indirect costs or that each Institute—rather than the grantee—reimburse NIDA for the cost of the cannabis.

3.   Non-NIH researchers - The subcommittee recommends that non-NIH researchers also be requested to reimburse NIDA for the cost of cannabis, as is possible. The subcommittee recognizes that NIDA will have to determine the availability of an appropriate mechanism for cost recovery from non federal entities.

OTHER CONSIDERATIONS: The subcommittee takes note that NIDA over the years has supported research on the clinical pharmacology of cannabis and recommends that NIDA now consider conducting research on the clinical pharmacology of cannabis at varied potencies and with different cannabinoid mixes.

Most clinical studies have been conducted using cannabis cigarettes with a potency of 2-4% THC. However, it is anticipated that there will be requests for cannabis cigarettes with a higher potency or with other mixes of cannabinoids. For example, NIDA has received a request for cigarettes with an 8% potency. The subcommittee notes that very little is known about the clinical pharmacology of this higher potency. Thus, while NIDA research has provided a large body of literature related to the clinical pharmacology of cannabis, research is still needed to establish the safety of new dosage forms and new formulations. Furthermore, drug interactions with other pharmaceuticals and alcohol have seldom been studied for any of the potencies. The subcommittee feels that it is within NIDA's purview to conduct research to address the clinical pharmacology and safety of cannabis and it recommends that NIDA continue to vigorously conduct this type of research.

‖ D

Appendix

Medical Organizations Supporting Supervised Access to Medical Marijuana

AIDS Action Council (1996)
AIDS Treatment News (1998)
Alaska Nurses Association (1998)
American Academy of Family Physicians (1995)
American Medical Student Association (1994)
American Preventive Medical Association (1997)
American Public Health Association (1994)
American Society of Addiction Medicine (1997)
Australian National Task Force on Cannabis (1994)
Being Alive: People With HIV/AIDS Action Committee (1996)
California Academy of Family Physicians (1994)
California Nurses Association (1995)
Colorado Nurses Association (1995)
Florida Medical Association (1997)
French Ministry of Health (1997)
Health Canada (1997)
Kaiser Permanente (1997)
Life Extension Foundation (1997)
Lymphoma Foundation of America (1997)
National Nurses Society on Addictions (1995)
New England Journal of Medicine (1997)
New York State Nurses Association (1995)
North Carolina Nurses Association (1996)
San Francisco Mayor's Summit on AIDS and HIV (1998)
Virginia Nurses Association (1994)

Medical Organizations Supporting
"Legal Access to Marijuana Under a Physician's Recommendation"

Alaska Nurses Association (1998)
California Academy of Family Physicians (1996)

California Nurses Association (1995)
Los Angeles County AIDS Commission (1996)
Maine AIDS Alliance (1997)
San Francisco Medical Society (1996)

Medical Organizations Supporting a Physician's Right to Recommend or Discuss Marijuana Therapy With a Patient

American Medical Association (1997)
American Society of Addiction Medicine (1997)
Bay Area Physicians for Human Rights (1997)
Being Alive: People With HIV/AIDS Action Committee (1997)
California Academy of Family Physicians (1997)
California Medical Association (1997)
Gay and Lesbian Medical Association (1997)
Marin Medical Society (1997)
San Francisco Medical Society (1997)

Medical Organizations Supporting Medical Marijuana "Research"

American Cancer Society (1997)
American Medical Association (1997)
American Public Health Association (1994)
American Society of Addiction Medicine (1997)
Australian National Task Force on Cannabis (1994)
British Medical Association (1997)
California Medical Association (1997)
California Society on Addiction Medicine (1997)
Congress of Nursing Practice (1996)
Federation of American Scientists (1994)
Florida Medical Association (1997)
Gay and Lesbian Medical Association (1995)
Health Canada (1997)
Kaiser Permanente (1997)
Lymphoma Foundation of America (1997)
NIH Workshop on the Medical Utility of Marijuana (1997)
National Nurses Society on Addictions (1995)
North Carolina Nurses Association (1996)
San Francisco Medical Society (1996)

Medical Organizations Supporting Other Favorable Positions Toward Medical Marijuana

British Medical Association (1997)–prescriptive access to active chemicals in marijuana; relaxation of present marijuana-law enforcement
California Medical Association (1998)–federal rescheduling
California Society on Addiction Medicine (1997)–federal rescheduling
Congress of Nursing Practice (1996)–instructing RN's on medical marijuana
New Mexico State Board of Nursing (1997)–endorsement of a RN's right to discuss marijuana therapy with a patient

Source: MarijuanaNews.Com

E

Appendix

Contact Information for Organizations that Support Medical Marijuana

Patients Out of Time

Tel: (434) 263-4484 / Fax: (434) 263-6753

E-mail: Patients@medicalcannabis.com / Website: www.medicalcannabis.com

Patients Out of Time is a national non-profit organization that was co-founded in 1995 by Al Byrne and Mary Lynn Mathre, R.N. The leadership of the organization is composed of health care professionals and experts in the clinical applications of cannabis and five of the remaining patients in the United States who receive their cannabis medicine from the federal government. All are volunteers.

National Organization for the Reformation of Marijuana Laws (NORML)

Tel: (202) 483-5500 / Fax: (202) 483-0057

E-mail: norml@norml.org / Website: www.norml.org

NORML is a nonprofit, public-interest lobby that for more than thirty years has provided a voice for those Americans who oppose marijuana prohibition. NORML represents the interests of the millions of Americans who smoke marijuana responsibly and believe the recreational and medicinal use of marijuana should no longer be a crime.

November Coalition

Tel: 509-684-1550

E-mail: moreinfo@november.org

Website: www.november.org

The November Coalition is a non-profit, grassroots organization that educates the public about the destructive increase in prison population in the United States due to current drug laws they feel are dangerous and wielded by a powerful federal authority acting far beyond its constitutional constraints.

Families Against Mandatory Minimums (FAMM)
Tel: (202) 822-6700 / Fax: (202) 822-6704
Website: www.famm.org

Families Against Mandatory Minimums is a national nonprofit organization founded in 1991 to challenge inflexible and excessive penalties required by mandatory sentencing laws. FAMM promotes sentencing policies that give judges the discretion to distinguish between defendants and sentence them according to their role in the offense, seriousness of the offense and potential for rehabilitation. FAMM's 25,000 members include prisoners and their families, attorneys, judges, criminal justice experts and concerned citizens. FAMM does not argue that crime should go unpunished, but that the punishment must fit the crime.

Fully Informed Jury Association (FIJA)
Tel: (406) 442-7800 / Fax: (406) 442-9332
Website: www.fija.org

A public policy, nonprofit educational foundation, FIJA's mission is to inform all Americans about their rights, powers and responsibilities when serving as trial jurors. FIJA also seeks to restore the political function of the jury as the final check and balance on our American system of government. FIJA programs and publications are possible because of contributions from individuals, foundations and corporations and through revenue generated from the sale of FIJA publications and materials.

American Civil Liberties Union (ACLU)
Website: www.aclu.org

The American Civil Liberties Union (ACLU) is our nation's guardian of liberty, working daily in courts, legislatures and communities to defend and preserve the individual rights and liberties guaranteed to all people in this country by the Constitution and laws of the United States.

Drug Policy Alliance
Tel: (212) 613-8020 / Fax: (212) 613-8021
Website: www.lindesmith.org

Drug Policy Alliance is the nation's leading organization working to end the war on drugs and promote new drug policies based on common sense, science, public health and human rights. The Alliance, headquartered in New York City, maintains offices in California, Washington, D.C., New Mexico and New Jersey.

Human Rights and the Drug War
Tel: (510) 215-8326
E-mail: mikki@hr95.org / Website: www.hr95.org/index.html

Human Rights and the Drug War is a multi-media project that combines the stories and photos of Drug War POWs with facts and figures about the US Drug War to confront the conscience of the American people and encourage individuals to take action for social justice.